Contents

Preface

Breast cancer is the most commonly diagnosed malignancy in women in Western countries, accounting for more than 178,000 cases in the US and more than 43,000 in the UK each year. Breast cancer accounts for as many diagnoses (26%) of cancer in US women as the second and third most common cancers: lung and bronchus (15%) and colorectal (11%). Major advances in the treatment of breast cancer have effected a reduction in the annual mortality in spite of the increasing incidence. Consequently, breast cancer accounts for 15% of cancer deaths in females in the US compared with 36% for lung and bronchus and colorectal cancer combined. This book describes the essentials of epidemiology, incidence, screening and pathology and the advances in treatment that have led to this improvement.

The main driver for the improvement in breast cancer outcomes has been high-quality clinical research. In the past, breast cancer clinical research was limited by fragmentation and lack of collaboration. During this period, progress was slow as small underpowered trials produced equivocal and/or conflicting results. The last decade has seen numerous large, often multinational, trials with rapid accrual and early results. The Breast International Group, founded in 1996 and chaired by Drs Martine Piccart and Aron Goldhirsch, has facilitated this collaboration of national and international research groups in breast cancer.

All aspects of breast cancer treatment have improved, from understanding the molecular subclassification, the routine histopathological description, diagnostic imaging, operations employed, treatments available and decision-making aids. There have been advances in endocrine therapy, chemotherapy and most notably biological target-directed therapy.

In postmenopausal women, aromatase inhibitors have become standard of care for the adjuvant treatment of steroid hormone receptor-positive breast cancer as a result of several large multinational trials. Anthracycline-based chemotherapy has become firmly established in the adjuvant arena and has been refined. Taxanes are routinely used in high-risk early breast cancer patients suitable for such therapy. The rapid development of HER-2-targeted therapy, from the description of the importance of this growth pathway by Slamon in 1987 to the adjuvant license within 20 years, represents the coming of age of translational research and rationale drug design. The efficacy of lapatinib after trastuzumab failure further illustrates the potential gain from the sequential targeting of a growth pathway that is fundamental to a

Dana-Farber Cancer Institute Handbook Series

Breast Cancer

rofessor of Medicine
Harvard Medical School,
Attending Physician
Gillette Center for Breast Oncology
Dana-Farber Cancer Institute
Department of Medicine, Brigham and Women's Hospital
Boston, MA, USA

Andrew Wardley
Consultant Oncologist
Medical Oncology Department
Christie Hospital NHS Trust
Manchester, UK

Series Editor
Arthur T. Skarin
Associate Professor of Medicine
Harvard Medical School
Senior Attending Physician
Medical Director, Lowe Center for Thoracic Oncology
Dana-Farber Cancer Institute
Department of Medicine, Brigham and Women's Hospital
Boston, MA, USA

MOSBY

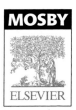

EDINBURGH LONDON NEW YORK OXFORD
PHILADELPHIA ST LOUIS SYDNEY TORONTO 2007

ELSEVIER
MOSBY

© 2003, Elsevier Limited.
© 2007 this compilation, Elsevier Limited. All rights reserved.

ISBN: 978 0 7234 3432 0

First published 2007
  Reprinted 2008

British Library Cataloguing in Publication Data
A catalogue record for this book is available from the British Library.

Library of Congress Cataloging in Publication Data
A catalog record for this book is available from the Library of Congress.

Note
Knowledge and best practice in this field are constantly changing. As new research and experience broaden our knowledge, changes in practice, treatment and drug therapy may become necessary or appropriate. Readers are advised to check the most current information provided (i) on procedures featured or (ii) by the manufacturer of each product to be administered, to verify the recommended dose or formula, the method and duration of administration, and contraindications. It is the responsibility of the practitioner, relying on their own experience and knowledge of the patient, to make diagnoses, to determine dosages and the best treatment for each individual patient, and to take all appropriate safety precautions. To the fullest extent of the law, neither the Publisher nor the Editors/Authors assume any liability for any injury and/or damage to persons or property arising out or related to any use of the material contained in this book.

The Publisher

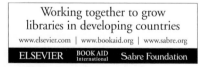

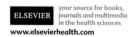

The
Publisher's
policy is to use
**paper manufactured
from sustainable forests**

Printed in China

particular cancer's growth. Other agents directed against elements within this pathway with possibly combination therapy is likely to lead to further patient benefits in a similar manner to that achieved by targeting the oestrogen receptor.

Screening has lead to a breast cancer population with a lower risk than was seen in the pre-screening era; this, together with better guidelines for the use of adjuvant systemic therapy, has resulted in a greater degree of overtreatment. Decision-making tools such as Adjuvant! Online are of considerable benefit with respect to helping patients decide whether or not to undertake additional treatment. Understanding resistance pathways and why current treatments fail holds the key to the future. Predictive biomarkers of sensitivity to specific treatments in individual patients with different types of breast cancer are required for tailoring treatment to the individual and improving cost-effectiveness.

This book provides a summary of the diagnosis, staging and treatment of patients with breast cancer and recent changes in treatment, as well as a pointer to future directions.

Andrew Wardley
Consultant Oncologist
Medical Oncology Department
Christie Hospital NHS Trust
Manchester, UK

Contributors

Susana M. Campos, MD MPH
Assistant Professor of Medicine
Harvard Medical School
Dana-Farber Cancer Institute
Department of Medicine
Brigham and Women's Hospital
Boston, MA, USA

Joseph P. Eder, MD
Assistant Professor of Medicine, Harvard Medical School
Phase I Group
Medical Oncology Division
Dana-Farber Cancer Institute
Department of Medicine
Brigham and Women's Hospital
Boston, MA, USA

Daniel F. Hayes, MD
Professor, Department of Internal Medicine
Co-Director, Breast Care Center
Clinical Director, Breast Cancer Program
University of Michigan
Ann Arbor, MI, USA

Janina A. Longtine, MD
Assistant Professor of Pathology, Harvard Medical School
Clinical Director, Molecular Biology Laboratory
Department of Pathology
Brigham and Women's Hospital
Boston, MA, USA

Tad Wieczorek, MD
Instructor in Pathology, Harvard Medical School
Department of Pathology
Brigham and Women's Hospital
Boston, MA, USA

Acknowledgements

The work of the associate editors of the *Atlas of Diagnostic Oncology* needs to be acknowledged. Dr Maxine Jochelson (currently Director of Oncologic Radiology and Women's Imaging, Cedars-Sinai Medical Center, Los Angeles, CA) and Dr Robert Penny (currently Director of Hematopathology, Community and St Vincent's Hospital of Indianapolis, IN) assisted with the first edition. Their immense help in organizing and evaluating the radiographic and pathology material for the chapters contributed significantly to the success of the *Atlas*. The work of the associate editors of the third edition, Dr Kitt Shaffer, currently Cambridge City Hospital, Cambridge, MA and Dr Tad Wieczorek, Instructor in Pathology at Brigham and Women's Hospital, is also deeply appreciated. Their expertise was invaluable in emphasizing the illustrative and teaching aspects of the third edition. Without their hard work on the *Atlas of Diagnostic Oncology* this Handbook would not have been possible.

Acknowledgement also has to go to the editorial staff at Elsevier Ltd for their assistance in preparing the *Dana-Farber Cancer Institute Handbook Series*.

The provision of figures to the *Atlas of Diagnostic Oncology* and the *Atlas of Breast Cancer* (Hayes, DF, ed.) that are reproduced in this Handbook is also acknowledged and appreciated.

Introduction

1

Arthur T. Skarin

As a result of improvements in healthcare and other factors, there is an increasing ageing population in the US and many other countries in the world. It has been estimated that the proportion of people over age 65 years of age will increase in the US from 12.6% in 2000 to 14.7% in 2015, and 20% in 2030.[1] This compares with 18.1% in Italy (used as a comparison as the oldest country in the world) in 2000, 22.2% in 2015, and 28.1% in 2030. Since the incidence of cancer increases with age, a rising number of cancer cases and deaths is predicted. Screening for cancer is therefore extremely important for early detection and subsequent cure. The annual screening recommendations by the American Cancer Society (ACS) have been updated recently,[2] and include clinical breast examination as part of a periodic health evaluation, preferably every 3 years under age 40 years and annually over age 40 years, and standard mammography beginning at age 40 years in asymptomatic women without a family history of breast cancer. Routine breast self-examination (BSE) has been de-emphasized because of the lack of strong evidence supporting its utility. Although BSE can increase awareness about breast changes, women should be informed about possible limitations and harms (e.g. false-positive results). For women who choose to do BSE, they should receive instruction and supervision regarding proper technique at the time of their periodic health exam. Recommendations for follow-up after diagnosis of breast cancer have been recently summarized.[3]

In the US, the likelihood of developing cancer during one's lifetime is approximately one in two for males and one in three for females, based on Surveillance, Epidemiology, and End Results data.[4] While the median age at cancer diagnosis is 68 years for men, it is 65 years for women. The overall 5-year relative survival rate for all patients is 65% with considerable variation by cancer site and stage at diagnosis. The variation in cancer statistics in males over recent years in the US is depicted in Figures 1.1 and 1.2. The ACS estimated that in 2006 the total number of new cases of cancer in women at all sites would be 679,510 with 273,560 deaths (see Figure 1.3).[4] The death rate from all cancers combined has decreased by 0.8% per year since 1992 for women. The mortality rate has continued to decrease for breast, and colon and rectum cancers in women. However, lung cancer deaths among women continue to increase slightly, paralleling the rise in cigarette smoking among women. Of interest, since 1999, cancer has surpassed heart disease as the leading cause of death for those under age 85 years; the reverse exists for those over age 85 years.[4]

Worldwide, an estimated 11 million new cases and 7 million cancer deaths occurred in 2002 while nearly 25 million people were living with cancer.[5] Global disparities in cancer incidence, mortality and prevalence relate to genetic susceptibility and ageing, but also to modifiable risk factors such as tobacco abuse, infectious agents, diet (low fruit and vegetable consumption) and physical activity. Other modifiable factors include overweight/obesity, urban air pollution, indoor smoke from household fires, unsafe sex, and contaminated injections in healthcare settings.[6] At least one-third of world cancer deaths are felt to be preventable. The associations of established causes of human cancers have been categorized as chemicals and naturally occurring compounds, medicines

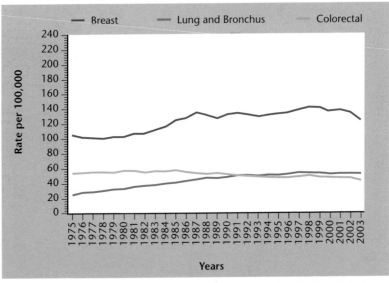

Fig. 1.1 Annual age-adjusted cancer incidence rates among females for selected cancers in the US, 1975 to 2002. Data from: Surveillance, Epidemiology, and End Results (SEER) program (http://seer.cancer.gov) SEER*Stat Database: Incidence – SEER 9 Regs Public-Use, Nov 2005 Sub (1973–2003), National Cancer Institute, DCCPS, Surveillance Research Program, Cancer Statistics Branch, released April 2006, based on the November 2005 submission.

and hormones, infectious agents and mixtures.[7] In breast cancer, only around 5–10% of cases are related to germline mutations inherited from a parent; mutations in *BRCA1* and/or *BRCA2* account for 50% of hereditary and familial breast cancers.[8]

Cancer prevention is extremely important and the progress in information technology has been recently reviewed.[9] Chemoprevention studies have been carried out for several cancers and have also recently been summarized.[10] Tamoxifen has been approved by the US Food and Drug Administration (FDA) for breast cancer prevention after 20 years of clinical research studies. This has been for both primary prevention in healthy women at higher breast cancer risk and secondary prevention of second primary breast cancers in women with a personal history of breast cancer.[10] Because of side effects from tamoxifen (mainly thromboembolic events and endometrial cancer) other newer agents and combinations of agents are under evaluation, including aromatase inhibitors and non-steroidal anti-inflammatory agents. Promising results have also been reported for the use of another selective oestrogen receptor modu-

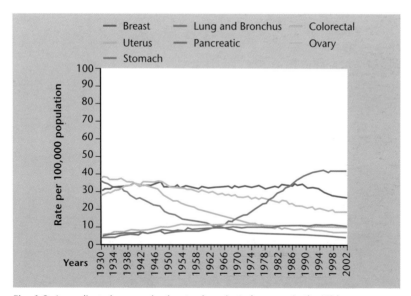

Fig. 1.2 Age-adjusted cancer death rates for selected cancers in the US between 1930 and 2002 for females. Source: US Mortality Public Use Data Tapes, 1960–2002, US Mortality Volumes, 1930–1959, National Center for Health Statistics, Centers for Disease Control and Prevention, 2005. Reproduced with permission from American Cancer Society. Cancer Facts and Figures 2006. Atlanta, American Cancer Society, Inc.

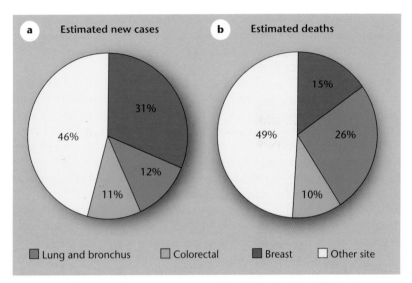

Fig. 1.3 Leading sites of new cancer cases and deaths in females – 2006 estimates. (a) Estimated new cases (b) Estimated deaths. Source: American Cancer Society, Inc., Surveillance Research. Estimates of new cases are based on incidence rates from 1979 to 2002, National Cancer Institute's Surveillance, Epidemiology, and End Results program, nine oldest registries. Estimates of deaths are based on data from US Mortality Public Use Data Tapes, 1969–2003, National Center for Health Statistics, Centers for Disease Control and Prevention, 2006.

lator, raloxifene, as a breast cancer chemoprevention agent.[11] Progress in chemoprevention drug development is rapid and has been recently reviewed in detail.[12] The goals are to integrate the specific molecular biomarker expressions into the development of new agents for chemoprevention of early intraepithelial neoplasia. The molecular targets summarized in this American Association for Cancer Research Task Force Report include anti-inflammatory/antioxidant agents, epigenetic modulation areas and signal transduction modulation targets. Six characteristics of neoplasms and the associated molecular targets that may be adversely affected by chemoprevention or definitive treatment programmes are noted in Table 1.1.[12]

With completion of the Human Genome Project new knowledge has become available about genetic variations to help elucidate possible genetic causes of cancer. Identification of mutations in genes may identify individuals at high risk for breast cancer (*BRCA1* and *BRCA2*, *p53*, *PTEN* and others) allowing for early detection, as well as furthering understanding of the aetiological subtypes of cancer and inherited alter-

Table 1.1 Molecular biomarkers associated with neoplasia characteristics[12]

Evading apoptosis
BCL-2, BAX, caspases, FAS, TNF receptor, DR5, IGF/PI3K/AKT, mTOR, p53, PTEN, *ras*, IL-3, NF-κB

Insensitivity to antigrowth signals
SMADs, pRb, cyclin-dependent kinases, MYC

Limitless replicative potential
hTERT, pRb, p53

Self-sufficiency in cell growth
Epidermal growth factor, platelet-derived growth factor, MAPK, PI3K

Sustained angiogenesis
VEGF, basic fibroblast growth factor, $\alpha_v\beta_3$, thrombospondin-1, hypoxia-inducible factor-1α

Tissue invasion and metastasis
Matrix metalloproteinases, MAPK, E-cadherin

BAX, BCL-2 associated X protein
BCL-2, B cell lymphoma 2
DR5, death receptor 5
FAS, fatty acid synthase
hTERT, human telomerase reverse transcriptase
IGF, insulin-like growth factor
IL, interleukin
MAPK, mitogen-activated protein kinase
mTOR, mammalian target of rapamycin
NF, nuclear factor
PI3K, phosphatidylinositol 3-kinase
pRb, retinoblastoma protein
PTEN, phosphatase and tensin homologue deleted on chromosome 10
TNF, tumour necrosis factor
VEGF, vascular endothelial growth factor

ations in drug metabolism. This exciting field of molecular epidemiology may thus impact favourably on cancer prognosis.[13] The importance of the above underscores the need for collection and storage of adequate tissue for study.

The new information explosion in molecular biology has led to important discoveries in unique patterns of gene expression characteristic of certain malignancies.[14] This genetic expression profiling will not only be important for accurate diagnosis but also for determining prognosis and candidates for certain therapies.[15] The results of these studies in breast cancer are encouraging, with favourable predictions of outcome.[16]

Another new blossoming area of research is cancer proteomics.[17] In this field, as the result of carcinogenesis, abnormalities in protein networks extend outside the cancer cell to the tissue microenvironment in which exchange of cytokines, enzymes and other proteins occurs to the advantage of the malignant cell. These molecules can be identified and become the target for new diagnostic and/or therapeutic targets. Major progress is occurring in the proteomics field in discovery of biomarkers that may be useful in prediction of clinical response to anticancer therapy.[18]

Major research advances have not only occurred during the past few years in cancer biology, genetic prevention and screening, but also in cancer treatment.[19] New standards of care for breast, lung, colon and other cancers became established during 2005. In breast cancer patients, several large randomized trials have revealed for the first time that adding trastuzumab (a targeted monoclonal antibody against the Her2neu protein) to standard chemotherapy in the adjuvant setting decreases the risk of recurrence by half and the risk of death by one-third compared with chemotherapy alone for patients with Her2neu-positive cancers.[19] The FDA indications for trastuzumab were recently expanded to include its use in early-stage breast cancer. There is also evidence of an increasing number of newer targeted therapies that can improve survival in some of the other common cancers. Targeted therapy has advantages of oral administration for many agents and directed attack on cancer cells, sparing most healthy cells including the hair and bone marrow. Other targeted therapies actively being investigated in breast cancer include those targeting endothelial growth factor receptor, vascular endothelial growth factor and other HER receptors. A detailed review of new and future therapeutic targets has been recently published.[20] Finally, multidisciplinary treatment guidelines from the National Comprehensive Cancer Network for breast cancer have been recently updated (www.nccn.org).

The *Dana-Farber Cancer Institute atlas of diagnostic oncology* was originally published in 1991 as a comprehensive reference and teaching aid in the various clinical, laboratory, pathological and radiological features of specific cancers. Because of the recent progress in understanding the molecular biology of cancer and the development of multiple chemotherapeutic agents it became apparent that there was a need for a combination of the teaching aspects of the *Atlas* with a review and recommendations of modern therapeutic programmes available to cancer patients. Thus arose the new *Dana-Farber Cancer Institute handbooks* of four common cancers – breast, colorectal, lung and prostate. Relevant sections of the 3rd edition of the *Atlas* have been updated and are now combined with a new chapter that includes treatment strategies.

In each of our *Handbooks* the authors will review important aspects of each cancer, including epidemiology, diagnostic work-up and staging evaluation, with photographic examples of pathology subtypes and clinical presentations, followed by an up-to-date detailed discussion of multimodality treatment programmes with current recommendations where necessary. In this book on breast cancer, Dr Wendy Chen, Attending Physician on the Breast Service at Dana-Farber Cancer Institute, reviews various aspects of comprehensive treatment including the use of new drugs and targeted agents. The importance of patient symptom management and quality of life efforts are also addressed.

REFERENCES

1. Yancik R: Population aging and cancer: a cross-national concern. Cancer J 2005; 11: 437–441.
2. Smith RA, Cokkinides V, Eyre HJ: American Cancer Society guidelines for the early detection of cancer, 2006. Cancer J Clin 2006; 56(1): 11–25.
3. Khatcheressian JL, Wolff AC, Smith TJ, et al: American Society of Clinical Oncology 2006 update of the breast cancer follow-up and management guidelines in the adjuvant setting. J Clin Oncol 2006; 24: 5091–5097.
4. Jemal A, Siegel R, Ward E, et al: Cancer statistics, 2006. CA Cancer J Clin 2006; 56: 106–130.
5. Kamangar F, Dores GM, Anderson WF: Patterns of cancer incidence, mortality, and prevalence across five continents: Defining priorities to reduce cancer disparities in different geographic regions of the world. J Clin Oncol 2006; 24(14); 2137–2150.
6. Ezzati M, Henley SJ, Lopez AD, Thun MJ: Role of smoking in global and regional cancer epidemiology: Current patterns and data needs. Int J Cancer 2005; 116: 963–971.
7. Neugent AI: Cancer epidemiology and prevention. Sci Am 2004; 12: 2–11.
8. Bennett IC, Gattas M, The BT: The management of familial breast cancer. Breast 2000; 9: 247–263.
9. Jimbo M, Nease DE, Ruffin MT, et al: Information technology and cancer prevention. CA Cancer J Clin 2006; 56: 26–36.
10. Tsao AS, Kim ES, Hong WK: Chemoprevention of cancer. Cancer J Clin 2004; 54: 150–180.
11. Vogel VG, Costantino JP, Wickerham DL, et al: Effects of tamoxifen vs raloxifene on the risk of developing invasive breast cancer and other disease outcomes: the NSABP Study of Tamoxifen and Raloxifene (STAR) P-2 trial. JAMA 2006; 295: 2727–2741.
12. Kelloff GJ, Lippman SM, Dannenberg AJ, et al: Progress in chemoprevention drug development: The promise of molecular biomarkers for prevention of intraepithelial neoplasia and cancer – a plan to move forward. Clin Cancer Res 2006; 12(12): 3661–3697.

13. Chen Y, Hunter DJ: Molecular epidemiology of cancer. Cancer J Clin 2005; 55(1): 45–54.
14. Ramaswamy S, Golub TR: DNA microarrays in clinical oncology. J Clin Oncol 2002; 20(7): 1932–1941.
15. Quackenbush J: Microarray analysis and tumor classification. N Engl J Med 2006; 354: 2463–2472.
16. Fan C, Oh D, Wessels L, et al: Concordance among gene-expression-based predictors for breast cancer. N Engl J Med 2006; 355: 560–569.
17. Geho DH, Petricoin EF, Liotta LA: Blasting into the microworld of tissue proteomics: A new window on cancer. Clin Cancer Research 2004; 10: 825–827.
18. Smith L, Lind MJ, Welham KJ, et al: Cancer proteomics and its application to discovery of therapy response markers in human cancer. Cancer 2006; 107(2): 232–241.
19. Herbst RS, Bajorin DF, Bleiberg H, et al: Clinical cancer advances 2005: Major research advances in cancer treatment, prevention, and screening – a report from the American Society of Clinical Oncology. J Clin Oncol 2006; 24(1): 190–205.
20. Von Hoff DD, Gray PJ, Dragovich T: Pursuing therapeutic targets that are and are not there: A tumor's context of vulnerability. Sem in Oncol 2006; 33(4): 367–368.

The role of molecular probes and other markers in the diagnosis and characterization of malignancy

2

Tad Wieczorek and Janina A. Longtine

Histopathological assessment is still the cornerstone in the diagnosis, classification and grading of malignancies. Light microscopic evaluation augmented by histochemical stains is sufficient in the majority of cases to provide adequate information for diagnosis and prognostication. However, it is limited by subjectivity and imprecision in the evaluation of poorly differentiated malignancies, tumours of unknown primary origin and unusual neoplasms. In an era of increasingly sophisticated therapeutic protocols (which sometimes target the molecular events leading to cancer) and the need to maximize information gained from minimally invasive samples (such as core biopsy or fine-needle aspiration), ancillary techniques have been developed to increase the specificity and reproducibility of diagnosis. These rely on cell-specific antigen expression and, more importantly, tumour-specific genetic changes that provide diagnostic, prognostic and/or therapeutic information.

In most instances, the advent of monoclonal antibodies directed against cellular proteins, coupled with the immunoperoxidase technique, has superseded direct ultrastructural evaluation in allowing more accurate designation of the epithelial, mesenchymal, haematolymphoid, neuroendocrine or glial origin of neoplasms. A cardinal example is immunolocalization of cytoskeletal intermediate filaments, which are differentially expressed in different cell types. Table 2.1 lists the intermediate filaments most useful in determining the cell lineage of tumours. The cytokeratins are a complex family of polypeptides that are expressed in various combinations in different epithelial cell types. Antibodies to cytokeratin subtypes can sometimes be utilized to identify the epithelial origin of a metastatic carcinoma of unknown primary site. For example, the pattern of reactivity for cytokeratin 7 (54 kD), which is expressed in most glandular and ductal epithelium and transitional epithelium of the urinary tract, and for cytokeratin 20 (46 kD), which is more restricted in its expression, has been helpful in this regard.[1]

In addition to the intermediate filaments, other monoclonal antibodies to cellular or tumour antigens are available. In the past decade, advances in the technique of immunohistochemistry have allowed

Table 2.1 Cytoskeletal intermediate filaments

Cell type	Intermediate filaments	Molecular weight or subtype	Presence in tumour
Epithelial	Cytokeratins	40–67	Keratinizing and non-keratinizing carcinomas
Mesenchymal	Vimentin	58	Wide distribution: sarcomas, melanomas, many lymphomas, some carcinomas
Muscle	Desmin	53	Leiomyosarcomas, rhabdomyosarcomas
Glial astrocytes	Glial fibrillary acidic protein	51	Gliomas (including astrocytomas), ependymomas
Neurons	Neurofilament proteins	68, 160, 200	Neural tumours, neuroblastomas

consistent, reliable application in routinely processed surgical pathology specimens.[2] Antigen retrieval techniques (including proteolytic digestion and heat-induced antigen retrieval), sensitive detection systems, automation and a broad range of antibodies have all contributed to this advance. Table 2.2 lists a panel of antibodies that can be utilized in routine formalin-fixed paraffin-embedded tissue to diagnose poorly differentiated neoplasms. A differential diagnosis is generated by clinical and morphological features, which can then be further refined by the use of immunohistochemistry. It is important to realize that the majority of antibodies are not entirely specific in lineage determination, and "aberrant" staining patterns are observed. In addition, there is biological variation in poorly differentiated neoplasms resulting in variation in protein expression. Therefore, accuracy is enhanced by using a panel of antisera to determine lineage or primary site. One application of this principle is distinguishing between poorly differentiated adenocarcinoma and mesothelioma in pleural tumours. Table 2.3 demonstrates the differential immunoprofile.

While a panel of monoclonal markers greatly aids in the diagnosis of a particular cancer, three malignancies can be confirmed solely by demonstrating the presence of a highly specific protein. Papillary and

Table 2.2 Immunocytochemistry in the differential diagnosis of malignancies

Malignancy	Keratin	Chromo-granin/ synaptophysin	S100	MART-1	LCA	OCT 3/4	SMA/ desmin
Carcinoma	+	–	–/+	–	–	–	–
Germ cell	+/–*	–	–	–	–	+/–	–
Lymphoma	–	–	–	–	+	–	–
Melanoma	–	–	+	+/–	–	–	–
Neuroendocrine	+/–	+	–	–	–	–	–
Sarcoma**	–/+	–	–/+	–/+	–	–	+/–

+ positive   +/– mainly positive, occasionally negative
– negative   –/+ mainly negative, occasionally positive

* Keratin is usually negative in seminomas, but positive in non-seminomatous germ cell tumours

**Sarcomas are a heterogeneous family of neoplasms and immunohistochemical staining patterns depend on the specific histological subtype

MART-1, Melanoma antigen recognized by T cells 1
LCA, Leukocyte common antigen
OCT3/4, Organic cation transporter 3/4
SMA, Smooth muscle actin

Table 2.3 Antibody panel in the differential diagnosis of adenocarcinoma and mesothelioma

Malignancy	Keratin*	WT-1	CD15 (Leu-M1)	CEA
Adenocarcinoma	+	–	+	+
Mesothelioma	+	+	–	–

*Keratin positivity in the appropriate clinicopathological setting limits the differential diagnosis to adenocarcinoma and mesothelioma

+ positive   – negative
CEA, carcinoembryonic antigen

follicular thyroid carcinomas are characterized by immunoreactivity to thyroglobulin, prostate carcinoma by detection of prostate-specific antigen, and breast carcinoma by a positive reaction for gross cystic disease fluid protein, which is present in approximately 50–70% of cases. It is noteworthy that the latter protein is also present in the rare apocrine gland carcinoma. Other antibodies which are not tissue-specific markers but useful in antibody panels include TTF-1 for pulmonary adenocarcinoma, RCC antigen for renal cell carcinoma, CD117 (c-kit) for gastrointestinal stromal tumours and CD31 (platelet endothelial cell adhesion molecule) for vascular endothelial neoplasms. Immunostains are also helpful in the delineation of normal tissue architecture and its abrogation in neoplasia. For example, immunostaining for p63 (a nuclear antigen expressed in myoepithelial cells of the breast and basal cells of the prostate) aids in the detection of ductal/glandular structures without the normal myoepithelial framework, the hallmark of invasive neoplasia.

While the cellular proteins expressed in particular types of neoplasia are fundamental to their diagnostic characterization, somatic mutations (i.e. mutations that occur in the genes of non-germline tissues) are central to the development of cancer. A series of different mutations in critical genes is probably necessary for malignant transformation to occur. The mutations may be deletions, duplications, point mutations and/or chromosomal translocations in the DNA of the tumour precursor cell. The mutations affect regulation of the cell cycle, differentiation, apoptosis, or cell–cell and cell–matrix interactions. Different neoplasms have different combinations of genetic alterations, which lead to clonal proliferations of cells. These genetic alterations, although fundamental in tumour biology, can also be used as diagnostic or prognostic markers for malignancies. This is best characterized in lymphomas and leukaemias where specific genetic translocations result in the production of chimeric mRNA and novel proteins. These translocations are the *sine qua non* for the classification of some leukaemias, such as the Philadelphia chromosome t(9;22)(q34;q11) for chronic myelogenous leukaemia and t(15;17)(q22;q11-21) for acute promyelocytic leukaemia.[3] Single nucleotide mutations may also be important in haematopoietic neoplasia; for example the *JAK2* V617F mutation is frequently present in chronic myeloproliferative disorders.[4] While genetic alterations in carcinomas are more complex than single point mutations or chromosome translocations, simple chromosomal translocations also commonly occur in (and characterize) soft tissue tumours.[5,6]

A global assessment of structural cytogenetic changes in a neoplasm is provided by full karyotypic analysis, which requires fresh, viable tumour. By contrast, fluorescence *in situ* hybridization (FISH) is a more targeted approach that can be performed on interphase nuclei obtained from frozen or fixed paraffin-embedded tissue and can identify specific characteristic cytogenetic abnormalities as an adjunct to tumour diagnosis. For example, FISH probes that flank the *EWS* gene region show a "split apart" signal when an *EWS* rearrangement is present, as in Ewing's sarcoma (see Figure 2.1). In addition, many of the characteristic cytogenetic abnormalities of neoplasms have been cloned and sequenced allowing for the utilization of molecular biology techniques such as Southern blot hybridization or, more commonly, the polymerase chain reaction (PCR). These techniques utilize fresh or frozen tumour, or even fixed, embedded tissue (with PCR), and improve diagnoses by identifying the characteristic chromosomal translocations of malignancies at the molecular level. With PCR, a specific translocation can be detected in as little as 1 in 100,000 or 1 in 1,000,000 cells as compared with 1 in 100 for FISH analysis. Thus, PCR provides a sensitive method for diagnosis and for monitoring response to therapy. For example, the t(9;22)(q34:q11) of chronic myelogenous leukaemia juxtaposes the *BCR* and *ABL1* genes resulting in a unique chimeric mRNA that can be detected by a quantitative real-time RT-PCR technique. Peripheral blood cell RNA is converted to cDNA by reverse transcription (RT). The resultant *BCR-ABL1* cDNA is quantified by monitoring fluorescently labelled oligonucleotide probes that specifically hybridize with the target during each cycle of PCR amplification (see Figure 2.2). Clinical trials with the tyrosine kinase inhibitor imatinib

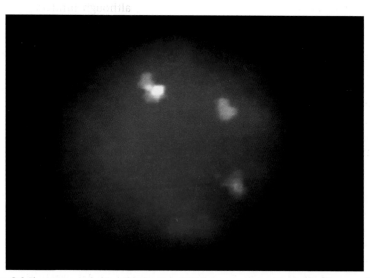

Fig. 2.1 Fluorescence *in situ* hybridization (FISH) on a sample obtained by fine-needle aspiration shows an interphase nucleus with red and green probes flanking each of two copies of the *EWS* gene, demonstrating one fused and one split signal. The split signal indicates rearrangement of the *EWS* gene region. (Courtesy of Dr. Paola Dal Cin, Cytogenetics Laboratory, Brigham and Women's Hospital.)

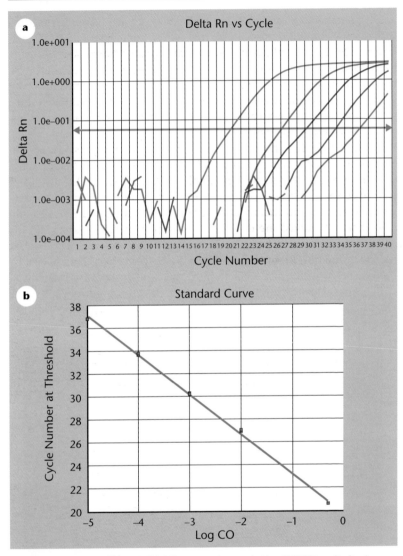

Fig. 2.2 (a) "Taq-Man™" (Applied Biosystems) quantitative RT-PCR results for dilutions (1:1,10^{-2}, 10^{-3}, 10^{-4}, 10^{-5}) of K562 cell line RNA which express chimeric *BCR-ABL1* mRNA. After approximately 15 cycles of PCR, the sample with the most *BCR-ABL1* mRNA (1:1) enters the linear phase of exponential amplification as measured by fluorescence accumulation monitored in real time. Samples with less target require more PCR cycles to reach the exponential phase. (b) For quantitation, a standard curve is generated plotting the PCR cycle number at threshold (red line in middle of exponential phase) against log concentration of target. Unknown samples can be quantified by plotting against the standard curve.

defined a target of a minimal residual level of *BCR-ABL1* RNA transcripts that is associated with progression-free survival (see Figure 2.3).[7,8] Rising levels of *BCR-ABL1* mRNA in patients on tyrosine kinase inhibitors or status post transplantation are indicative of a molecular relapse and the need for alternate or additional therapy. Southern blot hybridization or PCR can also identify clonal rearrangements of the immunoglobulin or T-cell receptor genes as an adjunct to the diagnosis of lymphoma or lymphoid leukaemias (see Figure 2.4).

Genetic analysis of neoplasms may also provide prognostic information, such as identifying the *BCR-ABL1* rearrangement in Philadelphia chromosome-positive acute lymphoblastic leukaemia (ALL) or *N-MYC* amplification in neuroblastoma. In addition, genetic analysis is playing an increasing role in therapeutic planning, as therapies tailored to specific genetic "lesions" are developed. Examples of such lesions include *HER2* amplification in breast cancer[9] and the epidermal growth factor receptor gene (*EGFR*) mutation in lung cancer.[10,11] These genetic lesions

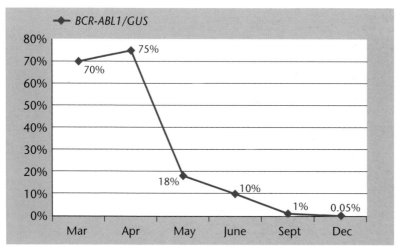

Fig. 2.3 Timeline of response to the tyrosine kinase inhibitor imatinib as monitored by real-time RT-PCR analysis of *BCR-ABL1* mRNA expressed as a ratio to the normalizing gene, *GUS*. Patients who achieve a 3-log reduction of transcript level by 12 months of therapy have a negligible risk of disease progression in the following 12 months.[8]

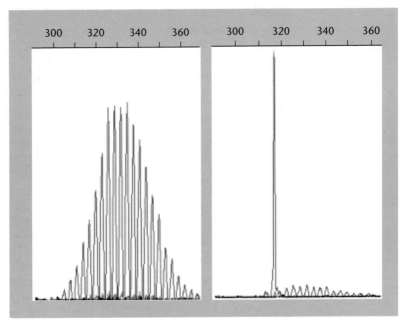

Fig. 2.4 Polymerase chain reaction (PCR) amplification of the immunoglobulin heavy chain (IgH) gene with primers to the variable and joining regions that flank the unique IgH gene rearrangement of B-cells. B-cell IgH rearrangements differ by size and sequence. Fluorescent primers are incorporated into the PCR product, which are then analyzed by capillary gel electrophoresis. (a) The Gaussian distribution of a polyclonal population of B cells. (b) A dominant peak of 318 bp representing a monoclonal population in a B-cell lymphoma.

may be detected either by evaluation of aberrant protein expression (as in immunohistochemical detection of membranous overexpression of HER2 oncoprotein in breast cancer), by gene amplification (as in FISH analysis of *HER2*), or by molecular testing (as in *EGFR* point or small deletion mutation analysis in lung cancer, see Figure 2.5). Quantification of the expression levels of large numbers of genes in specific types of neoplasia by oligonucleotide chips or cDNA microarrays, "expression profiling", has led to the identification of subsets of genes that provide prognostic information, such as in diffuse large B-cell lymphoma (see Figure 2.6).[12] It has even become feasible to measure the expression level of multiple genes (by RT-PCR) in routinely prepared, paraffin-embedded tumour samples, as in the multigene assay to

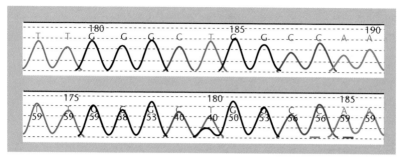

Fig. 2.5 Lung adenocarcinoma DNA sequence analysis of exon 21 of the *EGFR* receptor gene. The top row shows normal or wildtype exon sequence. The bottom row shows the heterozygous T to C point mutation, which characterizes the L858R mutation, a common mutation in carcinomas responsive to tyrosine kinase inhibitors.

predict recurrence of tamoxifen-treated, node-negative breast cancer.[13] This assay measures the expression level of genes involved in key aspects of tumour biology such as proliferation, invasion and oestrogen response and its quantitative result has potential application in therapeutic planning. As key genes (and hence proteins) are identified by expression profiling, expression can be assayed by routine immunohistochemistry. An important and practical example of this strategy was the development of a specific antibody to P504S (AMACR/racemase), a protein product strongly expressed in prostatic adenocarcinoma and prostatic intraepithelial neoplasia, but typically not in benign prostatic epithelium.[14] This immunostain is therefore useful in supporting a diagnosis of prostatic adenocarcinoma in cases where the morphological findings are subtle – as in the diagnosis of minimal adenocarcinoma on needle biopsy.

The genetics of cancer also extends to inherited predisposition to neoplasms described in a number of families.[15] These syndromes include germline mutations of tumour suppressor genes, such as familial retinoblastoma, and mutations of DNA repair genes as in ataxia-telangectasia or hereditary non-polyposis colon cancer. Some of these are listed in Table 2.4.

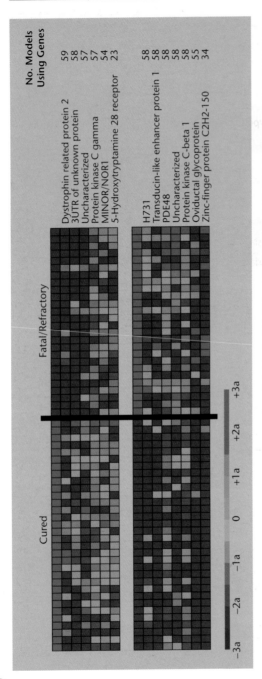

Fig. 2.6 Genes included in the DLBCL outcome model. Genes expressed at higher levels in cured disease are listed on top and those that were more abundant in fatal disease are shown on the bottom. Red indicates high expression; blue, low expression. Colour scale at bottom indicates relative expression in standard deviations from the mean. Each column is a sample, each row is a gene. Expression profiles of the 32 cured DLBCLs are on the left; profiles of the fatal/refractory tumours are on the right. Models with the highest accuracy were obtained using 13 genes. Reproduced by permission from Macmillan Publishers Ltd: Nature Medicine. Shipp M, Ross K, Tamayo P, et al: Diffuse large B-cell lymphoma outcome prediction by gene expression profiling and supervised machine learning. Nature Med 2002; 8: 68–74. © 2002.

Table 2.4 Examples of inherited syndromes predisposing to cancer

Syndrome	Chromosome locus	Gene
Ataxia-telangiactasia	11q22	ATM
Hereditary breast/ovarian cancer	17q21	BRCA1
	13q12	BRCA2
Familial adenomatous polyposis	5q21-q22	APC
Familial retinoblastoma	13q14	RB1
Hereditary non-polyposis colorectal cancer (Lynch syndrome)	2p22-p21	MSH2
	3p21	MLH1
	2q31-q33	PMS1
	7p22	PMS2
Li-Fraumeni	17p13	TP53
Multiple endocrine neoplasia, Type 1	11q13	MEN1
Multiple endocrine neoplasia, Type 2	10q11.2	RET
Neurofibromatosis, Type 1	17q11	NF1
Neurofibromatosis, Type 2	22q12	NF2
von Hippel-Lindau disease	3p26-p25	VHL

REFERENCES

1. Chu P, Wu E, Weiss LM: Cytokeratin 7 and cytokeratin 20 expression in epithelial neoplasms: a survey of 435 cases. Mod Pathol 2000; 13(9): 962–971.
2. Chan JKC: Advances in immunohistochemistry: Impact on surgical pathology practice. Seminars Diagn Pathol 2000; 17: 170–177.
3. Jaffe ES, Stein HN, Vardiman JW, eds: World Health Organization Classification of Tumours, Pathology and Genetics of Tumours of Haematopoietic and Lymphoid Tissues. IARC Press, Lyon, 2001.
4. Percy MJ, McMullin MF: The V617F JAK2 mutation and the myeloproliferative disorders. Hematol Oncol 2005; 23(3-4): 91–93.
5. Sandberg AA: Cytogenetics and molecular genetics of bone and soft-tissue tumors. Am J Med Genet 2002; 115(3): 189–193.
6. Antonescu CR: The role of genetic testing in soft tissue sarcoma. Histopathology 2006; 48(1): 13–21.
7. O'Brien SG, Guilhot F, Larson RA, et al: Imatinib compared with interferon and low-dose cytarabine for newly diagnosed chronic-phase chronic myeloid leukemia. N Engl J Med 2003; 348: 994–1004.
8. Hughes TP, Kaeda J, Branford S, et al: Frequency of major molecular responses to imatinib or interferon alfa plus cytarabine in newly diagnosed chronic myeloid leukemia. N Engl J Med 2003; 349: 1423–1432.

9. Slamon DJ, Leyland-Jones B, Shak S, et al: Use of chemotherapy plus a monoclonal antibody against HER2 for metastatic breast cancer that overexpresses HER2. N Engl J Med 2001; 344: 783–792.

10. Lynch TJ, Bell DW, Sordella R, et al: Activating mutations in the epidermal growth factor receptor underlying responsiveness of non-small-cell lung cancer to gefitinib. N Engl J Med 2004; 350: 2129–2139.

11. Paez JG, Janne PA, Lee JC, et al: EGFR mutations in lung cancer: correlation with clinical response to gefitinib therapy. Science 2004; 304: 1497–1500.

12. Shipp M, Ross K, Tamayo P, et al: Diffuse large B-cell lymphoma outcome prediction by gene expression profiling and supervised machine learning. Nature Med 2002; 8: 68–74.

13. Paik S, Shak S, Tang G, et al: A multigene assay to predict recurrence of tamoxifen-treated, node-negative breast cancer. N Engl J Med 2004; 351: 2817–2826.

14. Beach R, Gown AM, De Peralta-Venturina MN, et al: P504S immunohistochemical detection in 405 prostatic specimens including 376 18-gauge needle biopsies. Am J Surg Pathol 2002; 26(12): 1588–1596.

15. Scriver CR, Beaudet AL, Sly WS, Valle D, eds: Metabolic and Molecular Bases of Inherited Disease, 8th edn. McGraw-Hill, New York, 2001.

Breast cancer: epidemiology, histology, diagnosis and staging

3

Susana M. Campos, Daniel F. Hayes, Wendy Y. Chen

INTRODUCTION

Breast cancer is a major cause of morbidity and mortality in women over 45 years of age, especially in the US. In 2007, it is estimated that over 178,000 new cases will be diagnosed and more than 40,000 women will die of the disease in the US. Overall, mortality due to breast cancer has been declining in the western world over the last two decades. It is a highly heterogeneous disease, both pathologically and clinically. Although age is the single most common risk factor for the development of breast cancer in women (see Figure 3.1),

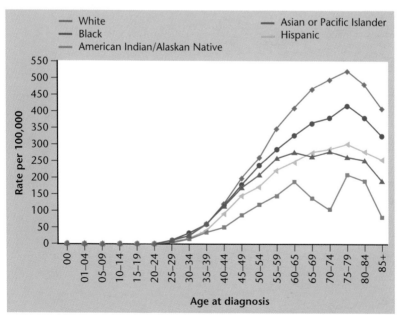

Fig. 3.1 Age-incidence curve for breast cancer. Data from Surveillance, Epidemiology, and End Results (SEER) Program (http://seer.cancer.gov) SEER*Stat Database: Incidence – SEER 13 Regs Public-Use, Nov 2005 Sub (1992–2003), National Cancer Institute, DCCPS, Surveillance Research Program, Cancer Statistics Branch, released April 2006, based on the November 2005 submission.

many other epidemiological associations have been identified. These include a germline mutation in *BRCA1* or *BRCA2*, family history of breast cancer, a prior history of breast cancer, early menarche, late age at first full-term pregnancy, personal history of benign breast disease, hormone replacement therapy and several lifestyle factors (see Table 3.1). It should be noted that there is also significant geographical variation in breast cancer rates (see Figure 3.2).

Table 3.1 Selected breast cancer risk factors

Risk factor	Referent	Comparison	Approximate relative risk	Selected references
Age (years)	See Figure 3.1			
Age at menarche	>14 years	<12 years	1.2–1.5	1–3
Oral contraceptive use	None	Current	1.1–1.2	4,5
Age at first birth	<20–22 years	>28–35 years	1.3–1.8	2,3,6
Breast feeding	None	12 months	0.9	7
Parity	0	5+	0.6	2
Age at menopause				
Surgical oophorectomy	50+ years	<40 years	0.6	1
Oestrogen + progestogen	None	Current use for 5 years	1.2–1.3	8
Body mass index				
Premenopausal	<21 kg/m²	>31 kg/m²	0.5–0.7	9,10
Postmenopausal	<21 kg/m²	>28–30 kg/m²	1.2–1.3	10
Physical activity	None	Moderate	0.6–0.9	11,12
Serum oestradiol (postmenopausal)	Lowest quartile	Highest quartile	2	13
Mammographic breast density	<25% density	>75% density	4–6	14
Bone density	Lowest quartile	Highest quartile	2.0–3.5	15,16
Alcohol consumption	None	3+ drinks per day	1.3–1.4	17,18
Benign breast disease (atypical hyperplasia)	No	Yes	2–6	19,20
Family history of breast cancer in first-degree relative	None	1+	2–4	21

Much progress has been made in the diagnosis and treatment of primary and metastatic breast cancer in the last 20 years. The widespread use of routine mammography has led to increased detection of early primary lesions, a factor that has contributed to a significant decrease in mortality (see Figures 3.3–3.7). Magnetic resonance imaging (MRI) of the breast has been useful in detecting smaller lesions not identified by either modality but its specificity is less than that for mammography (see Figure 3.8). Moreover, less aggressive, conservative local therapy has been shown to be as effective as mastectomy in prolonging survival, while avoiding the cosmetic disfigurement associated with more extensive surgery. Sentinel node biopsy (see Figure 3.9) has decreased the morbidity associated with the traditional axillary node dissection. Adjuvant systemic therapy, such as chemotherapy and/or hormonal

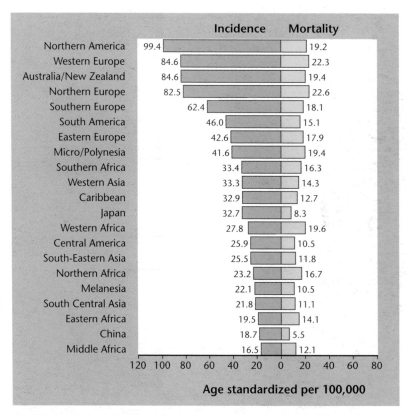

	Incidence	Mortality
Northern America	99.4	19.2
Western Europe	84.6	22.3
Australia/New Zealand	84.6	19.4
Northern Europe	82.5	22.6
Southern Europe	62.4	18.1
South America	46.0	15.1
Eastern Europe	42.6	17.9
Micro/Polynesia	41.6	19.4
Southern Africa	33.4	16.3
Western Asia	33.3	14.3
Caribbean	32.9	12.7
Japan	32.7	8.3
Western Africa	27.8	19.6
Central America	25.9	10.5
South-Eastern Asia	25.5	11.8
Northern Africa	23.2	16.7
Melanesia	22.1	10.5
South Central Asia	21.8	11.1
Eastern Africa	19.5	14.1
China	18.7	5.5
Middle Africa	16.5	12.1

Age standardized per 100,000

Fig. 3.2 Breast cancer incidence by geographic area. Reproduced with permission from Parkin DM, Bray F, Ferlay J, Pisani P. Global cancer statistics, 2002. CA Cancer J Clin 2005; 55: 74–108. © American Cancer Society.

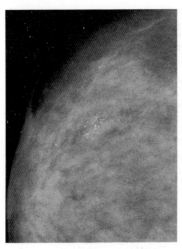

Fig. 3.3 Stage I (T1N0) breast cancer. Magnified view of a screening mammogram from a 52-year-old woman who had no palpable mass demonstrates the classic clustered microcalcifications of several shapes and sizes highly suggestive of carcinoma. Some exhibit linear branching, which is even more suggestive of a ductal lesion. Biopsy confirmed an early invasive ductal carcinoma. (Courtesy of Dr P. Stomper, Roswell Park Memorial Institute, Buffalo, NY, USA.)

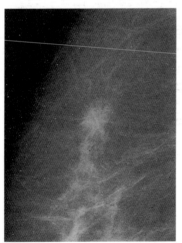

Fig. 3.4 Stage (T1N0) breast cancer. Magnified view of a mammogram from a 50-year-old woman with a history of 'lumpy' breasts shows a 1.0 cm stellate mass in the superior portion of the breast. The lesion was excised and found to be an invasive ductal carcinoma. (Courtesy of Dr P. Stomper, Roswell Park Memorial Institute, Buffalo, NY, USA.)

therapy, has also contributed to the prolonged survival of patients with early breast cancer. Finally, the identification of molecular targets such as the over-expression of Her2neu has led to the incorporation of biological therapy in both the adjuvant and metastatic settings resulting in improved survival for Her2neu-positive cancers.

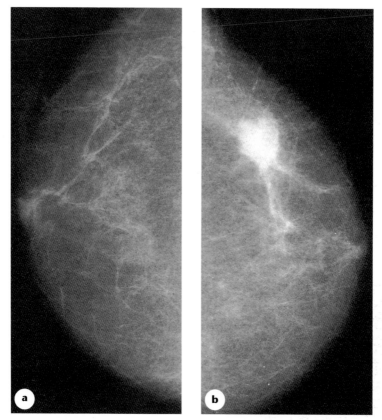

Fig. 3.5 Stage IIA (T2N0) breast cancer. This mammogram from a 65-year-old woman shows that the breasts are not too dense (**a**); therefore, the 2.5 cm stellate mass in the upper outer quadrant of the right breast was easily palpated (**b**). Histological examination following resection showed an invasive ductal carcinoma.

INCIDENCE

Breast cancer incidence rates have remained level during the last decade. Breast cancer deaths are decreasing, primarily for white women and younger women. Although white women develop breast cancer more frequently, black women are more likely to die of the disease.

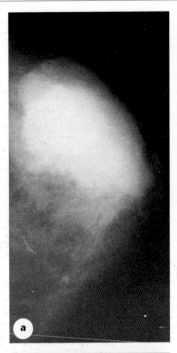

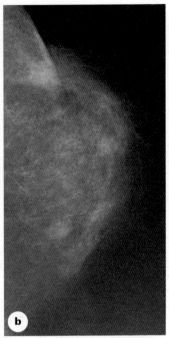

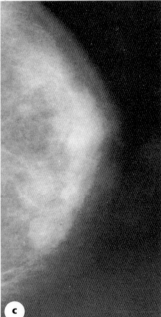

Fig. 3.6 Stage IIIB (T4N0) breast cancer. A 45-year-old woman presented with a very large (10 cm) primary tumour. There was an inflammatory component, but a distinct underlying mass was palpable and quite easily detected on the mammogram (**a**). (**b**) Following chemotherapy and radiotherapy, the mass completely disappeared, replaced only by the distortion artefact left by the biopsy. Three months later, the tumour recurred within the same breast. (**c**) The mammogram demonstrates multiple nodular tumour masses.

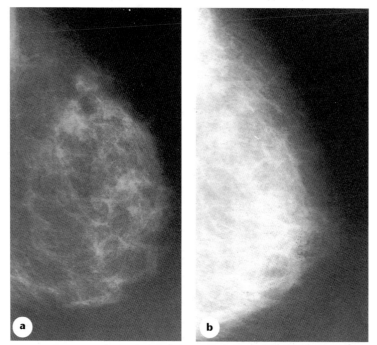

Fig. 3.7 Stage IIB (T4) breast cancer. Seven months after a normal baseline mammogram (**a**), a 35-year-old woman developed skin thickening and erythema of the breast. (**b**) At that time, her mammogram demonstrated a diffuse increase in density – a characteristic finding in inflammatory breast cancer corresponding to the lack of a distinct mass. Biopsy confirmed the diagnosis of inflammatory breast cancer.

SCREENING

Routine mammographic screening allows better detection of primary breast cancers than physical examination. Mammographic screening has been shown to decrease mortality rates in women 50–69 years of age. A 26% decrease in the relative risk of breast cancer was noted with screening mammography in this group. The role of screening mammography in women 40–49 years of age remains controversial. Current imaging modalities include mammography, ultrasound and, recently, MRI. Only mammography has been demonstrated to be a valuable tool and associated with a decrease in breast cancer mortality in randomized trials.

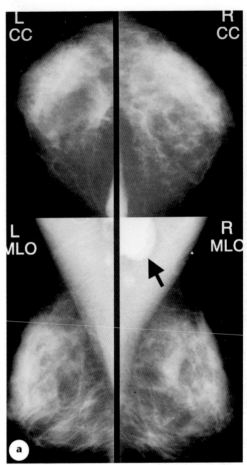

Fig. 3.8 (a) Bilateral mammograms on a 45-year-old patient with enlarged right axillary nodes (black arrow) but no mammographic abnormality within either breast.

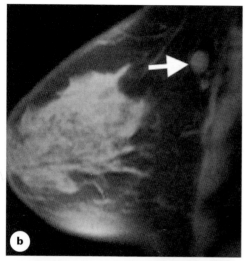

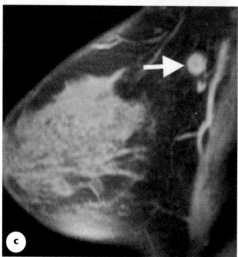

(b) Sagittal magnetic resonance (MR) image of the right breast with fat saturation prior to administration of gadolinium. A rounded density represents an axillary node (white arrow). (c) Sagittal MR image at the same location as (b) after administration of gadolinium. Enhancement of the node is evident (white arrow).

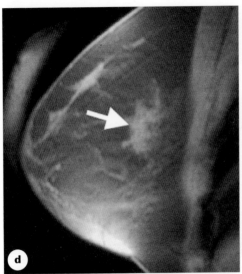

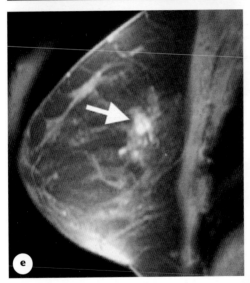

Fig. 3.8 *Continued* (d) Sagittal MR image of the right breast at a level slightly medial to (b) and (c). A patch of stromal density is evident deep in the breast prior to contrast administration (white arrow). Other retroareolar stromal densities with similar appearance are also present. (e) Sagittal MR image of the right breast in the same location as (d), after administration of gadolinium. The deep stroma is enhancing (white arrow) consistent with tumour, while the other stromal densities have not changed, consistent with normal breast tissue.

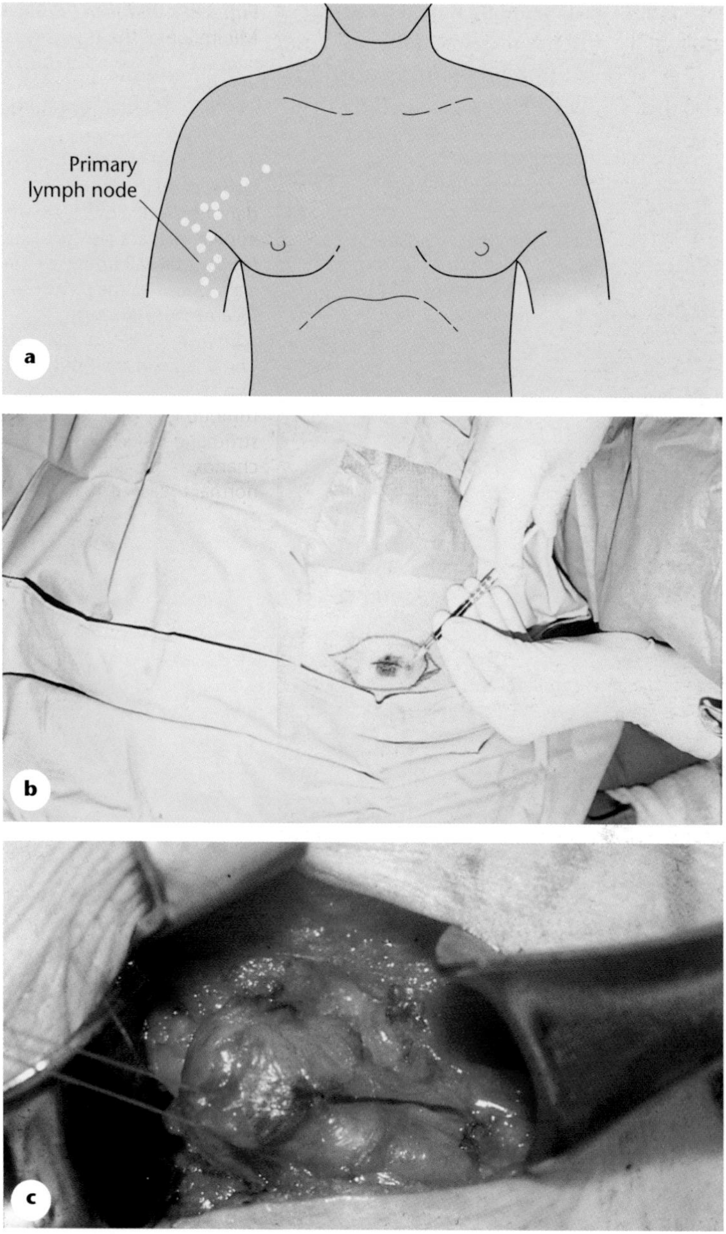

Fig. 3.9 Sentinel node biopsy. (a) Axillary lymph mapping. (b) Injection of blue dye in the tumour cavity. (c) Identification of the sentinel node (follow blue line).

Over half of all women will develop benign breast lesions. These include macro- and microcysts, adenosis, apocrine changes, intraductal papillomas, fibrosis, fibroadenomas and epithelial hyperplasias (see Figures 3.10–3.18). Only the latter, particularly those showing dysplastic changes,

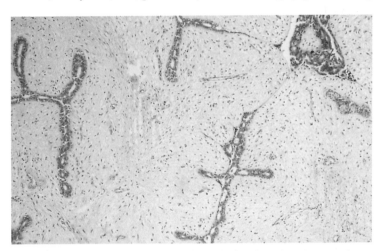

Fig. 3.10 Fibroadenoma. The tumour from which this histological section was taken was a well-circumscribed, discoid mass, clearly demarcated from the surrounding breast tissue. High magnification reveals stroma compressing the ducts so that they form slit-like curvilinear spaces. Note the low cellularity of the stroma, an important benign feature.

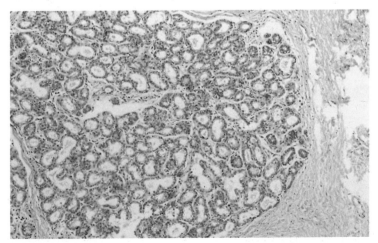

Fig. 3.11 Lactating adenoma. This well-circumscribed lesion has closely packed acini with prominent epithelial cells marked by large nuclei and abundant, pink, vacuolated cytoplasm. (Courtesy of Dr N. Weidner, Brigham and Women's Hospital, Boston, MA, USA.)

are believed to be precursors to the development of malignancy. Benign lesions may present with pain, tenderness and nipple discharge, as well as masses and dimpling of the skin. Mammographic changes such as densities and microcalcifications are also noted in benign lesions. They may mimic malignancies.

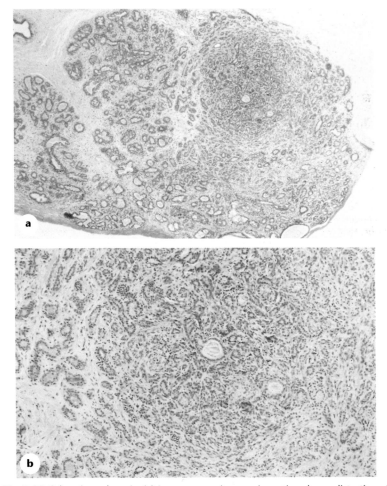

Fig. 3.12 Sclerosing adenosis. (**a**) Low-power microscopic section shows distortion of the lobular architecture; there is an increase in acini (terminal ductules), appearing in a whorled, expansile and vaguely defined pattern. The low-power view is very helpful in distinguishing this benign proliferation from malignancy. (**b**) Higher magnification shows that the acini are composed of a normal two-cell population.

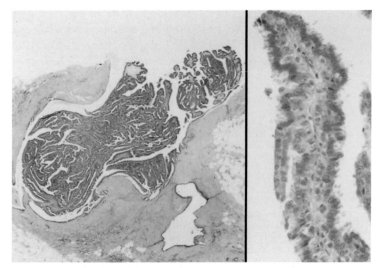

Fig. 3.13 Papilloma. Low-magnification view shows a large duct filled with a papillary proliferation. At higher power (inset), a papillary branch can be seen with a normal two-cell population covering a fibrovascular stalk. In this benign tumour, the lining epithelial cells can exhibit apocrine changes.

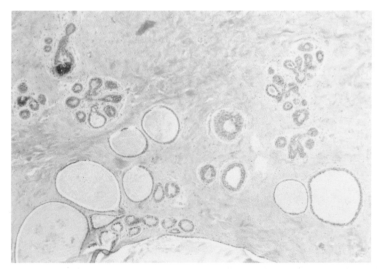

Fig. 3.14 Fibrocystic changes. These benign changes are the most common findings in breast biopsies. They are characterized by dense fibrosis intermixed with cystic areas.

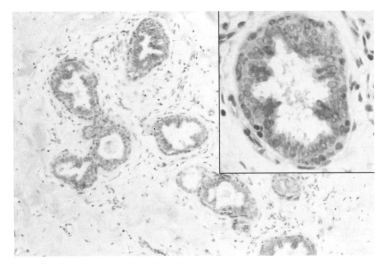

Fig. 3.15 Epithelial hyperplasia (mild). This lobular unit exhibits irregular areas of heaped-up cells lining the acini (terminal ductules). At high magnification (inset), the epithelial layer of one ductule is 3–4 cell layers thick and there is no bridging of cells across the acinar structure.

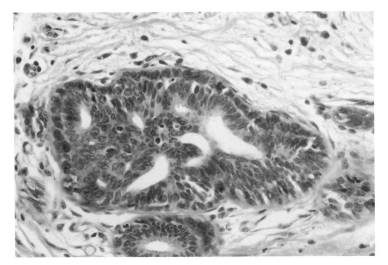

Fig. 3.16 Epithelial hyperplasia (moderate). At this stage, the acinar structure is distended by hyperplastic cells that frequently bridge the lumen, often filling as much as half of it.

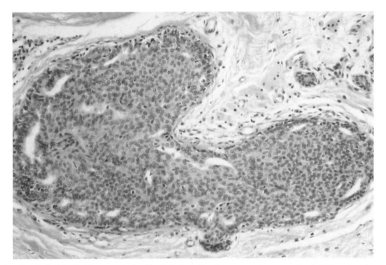

Fig. 3.17 Epithelial hyperplasia (florid). Involved spaces show marked distension by hyperplastic cells that occupy the majority of the lumen. Collapsed slit-like spaces are present, frequently at the periphery of the structure. These slits are surrounded by serpentine passages composed of 'flowing' cells, which often lack clear cell borders. Moderate and florid hyperplasias imply a slightly higher risk of subsequent invasive carcinoma than mild or no hyperplasia.

HISTOLOGY

IN SITU BREAST CANCERS/NON-INVASIVE BREAST CANCER

The enthusiasm for screening has led to the detection of small primary lesions that pose difficult diagnostic dilemmas when breast biopsies reveal premalignant histopathological findings. The diagnosis of *in situ* carcinomas appears to be increasing in frequency. Non-invasive breast cancer includes ductal carcinoma *in situ* (DCIS) and lobular carcinoma *in situ* (LCIS). DCIS is described as the proliferation of malignant epithelial cells confined to the mammary ducts without evidence of invasion through the basement membrane (see Figures 3.19–3.24). It is considered a precursor lesion. DCIS (also called intraductal carcinoma) is more likely to be localized to a region within one breast. Variants include papillary carcinoma *in situ* (see Figure 3.25), which may mimic benign atypical papillomatosis, and comedo carcinoma, which consists of a solid growth of neoplastic cells within the ducts, associated with centrally located necrotic debris.

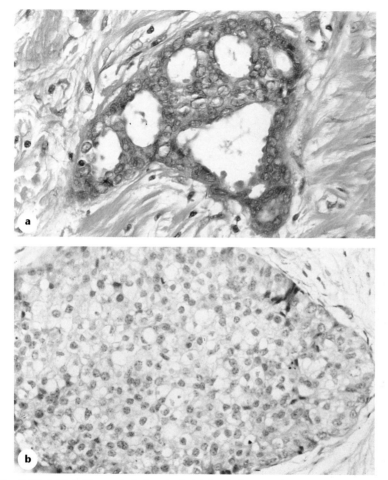

Fig. 3.18 Epithelial hyperplasia (atypical). **(a)** Atypical cases exhibit a non-uniform population of cells from normochromatic nuclei surrounding spaces that are not quite smooth-lined. It is these features that distinguish atypical epithelial (ductal) hyperplasia from ductal carcinoma *in situ*, in which smooth, geometric spaces are surrounded by a uniform cell population with hyperchromatic nuclei. **(b)** High magnification shows that these proliferating, relatively non-uniform cells lack the necessary degree of cell-to-cell rigidity. Atypical hyperplasia carries a relatively higher risk of subsequent development of invasive carcinoma than other types. This risk is further elevated in women with a family history of breast cancer in a first-degree relative.

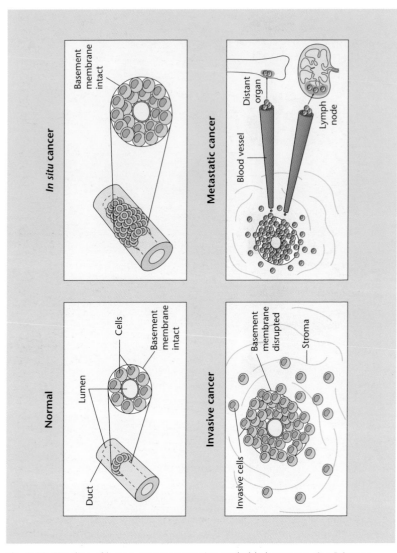

Fig. 3.19 Timeline of breast cancer suggesting probable heterogeneity. Primary breast cancers begin as single (or more) cells that have lost normal regulation of differentiation and proliferation but remain confined within the basement membrane of the duct or lobule. As these cells go through several doublings, at some point they invade through the basement membrane of the ductule or lobule and ultimately metastasize to distant organs.

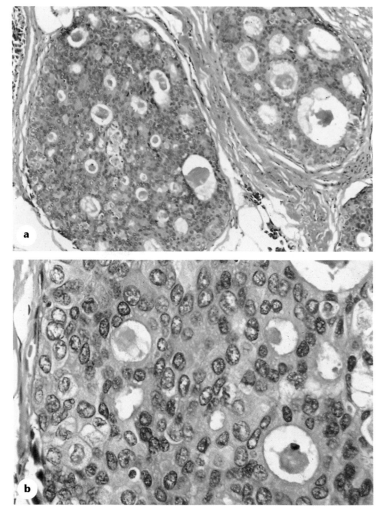

Fig. 3.20 Intraductal carcinoma (cribriform type). (a) Low- and (b) high-power photomicrographs demonstrate a cribriform pattern composed of a rather uniform tumour cell population with distinct cytoplasmic borders; the cells are rigidly arranged around crisp, circular holes. With this pattern, the risk for the subsequent development of invasive cancer increases 10–11-fold. (Courtesy of Dr N. Weidner, Brigham and Women's Hospital, Boston, MA, USA.)

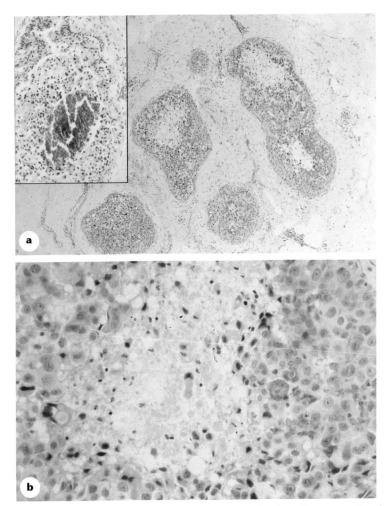

Fig. 3.21 Intraductal carcinoma (comedo type). (**a**) Low- and medium-power (inset) microscopic sections show expanded ducts with central necrosis. (**b**) At high magnification, cellular pleomorphism is also evident. This feature is seen to a greater extent and more commonly in the comedo type of ductal carcinoma *in situ*. Occult invasive elements may also be more common in the comedo than non-comedo types (see Figures 3.22, 3.23 and 3.25).

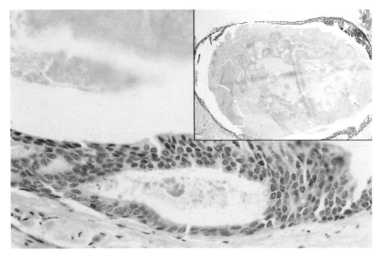

Fig. 3.22 Intraductal carcinoma ('clinging' type). Low- (inset) and high-power microscopic sections show tumour cells 'clinging' to the periphery of a duct. The clusters of basophilic malignant cells exhibit a high nucleus-to-cytoplasm ratio. Note the bridge-like structure formed by these cells on the high-power view.

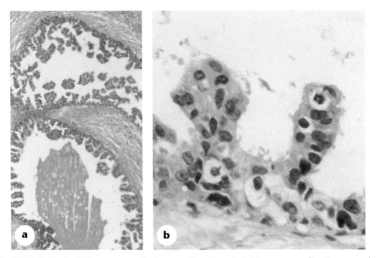

Fig. 3.23 Intraductal carcinoma (micropapillary type). (**a**) Low magnification reveals expanded ducts with fronds of tumour characteristically extending toward the centre of the lumina. (**b**) At high magnification, the bulbous fronds typically appear narrow at the base and expanded at the tip. (**a**: Courtesy of Dr N. Weidner, Brigham and Women's Hospital, Boston, MA, USA.)

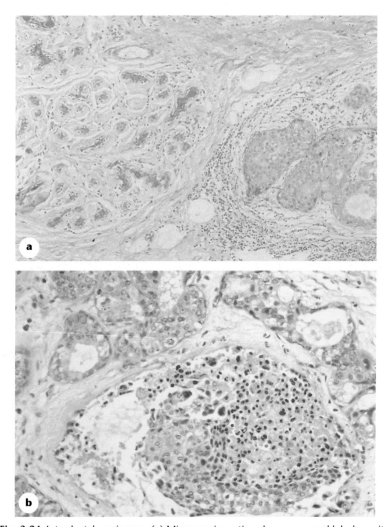

Fig. 3.24 Intraductal carcinoma. (**a**) Microscopic section shows a normal lobular unit on the left and 'cancerization of the lobules' on the right, where a ductal carcinoma has extended into the lobules. (**b**) High magnification demonstrates 'cancerization of the lobules' in the upper portion of the field, while the lower portion reveals a duct that has been expanded by an intraductal carcinoma with foci of necrosis.
'Cancerization of the lobules' carries no clinical significance except that it may mimic lobular carcinoma *in situ*. However, pleomorphism, tubule formation and necrosis, as seen here, are not encountered in lobular carcinoma.

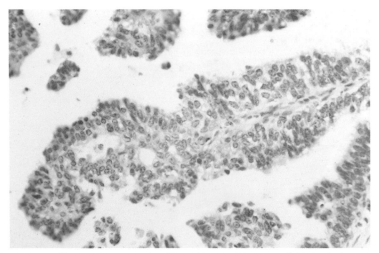

Fig. 3.25 Papillary carcinoma *in situ*. The architectural features of this *in situ* breast cancer are similar to those of a papilloma. The normal two-cell-layer epithelium covering the fibrovascular fronds is replaced by a uniform proliferation of cells with hyperchromatic nuclei.

In contrast, LCIS (see Figures 3.26 and 3.27) tends to be diffusely distributed throughout both breasts. LCIS is considered a risk factor for breast cancer and is not a precursor lesion.

Intraductal carcinoma is more common than LCIS, representing about 21% of cases of breast cancer diagnosed in the US. Please see Chapter 4 for information on the treatment of DCIS and LCIS.

INVASIVE BREAST CANCERS

Over 75% of all infiltrating breast cancers originate in the ductal system (see Figures 3.28–3.31 and Table 3.2). A number of histological variants of ductal carcinoma have been described. Pure examples of these variants constitute only a small percentage of the total number of cases, but certain features of each may be seen within the main portions of tumours that exhibit the more common presentation designated as invasive (or infiltrating) ductal carcinoma. Medullary carcinoma (see Figure 3.32) is distinguished by poorly differentiated nuclei and infiltration by lymphocytes and plasma cells, while tubular carcinomas (see Figure 3.33) are

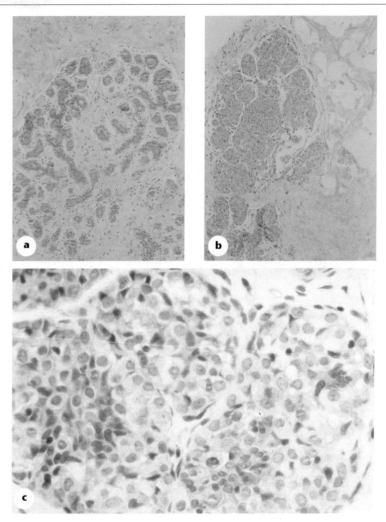

Fig. 3.26 Lobular carcinoma *in situ* (LCIS). Low-power photomicrographs show (**a**) the normal architecture of a lobular unit and (**b**) a distended lobular unit exhibiting the typical appearance of LCIS. (**c**) At high magnification, the lobular unit is seen to be distended and distorted by characteristically uniform, round tumour cells with bland nuclei. LCIS is usually diffusely dispersed throughout the breast and is often bilateral. Rarely producing a mass or abnormality on mammography, it is commonly discovered coincidentally during a biopsy performed for other suspicious lesions. Women with LCIS have a slightly higher risk of developing invasive cancer, whether ductal or lobular in origin, in their lifetime.

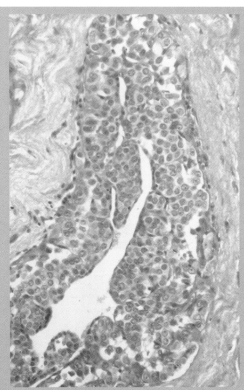

Fig. 3.27 Lobular carcinoma *in situ*. High-power microscopic section shows clusters of tumour cells spreading along a duct in a 'pagetoid' fashion; that is, displacing the normal ductal epithelium toward the lumen, which is lined by attenuated luminal surface cells. This should not be confused with Paget's disease of the breast, a lesion of ductal origin, in which tumour cells extend into the epidermis.

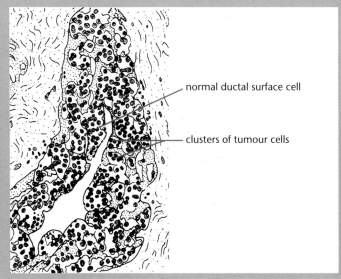

normal ductal surface cell

clusters of tumour cells

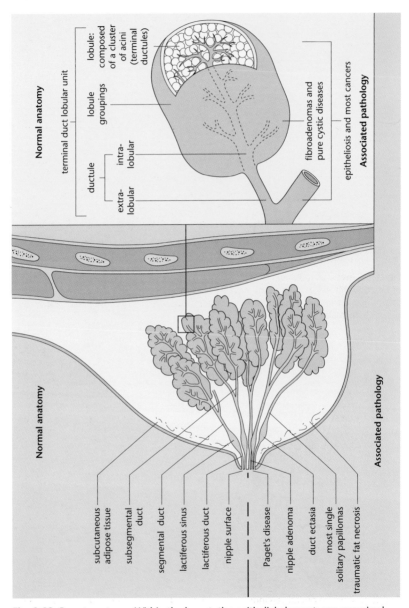

Fig. 3.28 Breast anatomy. Within the breast, the epithelial elements are organized into lobular units consisting of acini that feed into ductules. The latter in turn coalesce into larger ducts that form a reservoir, or lactiferous sinus, proximal to the nipple. These epithelial structures, supported by adipose and fibrous tissue, give rise to more than 95% of breast malignancies.

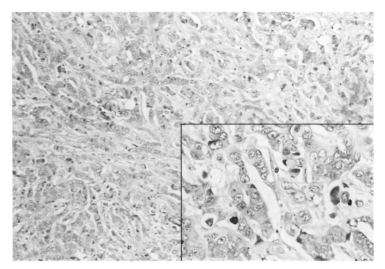

Fig. 3.29 Invasive ductal carcinoma. Low- and high-power (inset) photomicrographs of a poorly differentiated adenocarcinoma show that the stroma is infiltrated by pleomorphic tumour cells exhibiting a high mitotic rate. Note the necrosis and lack of tubule formation.

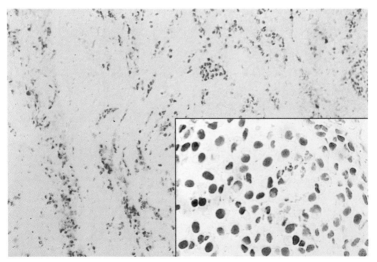

Fig. 3.30 Invasive ductal carcinoma. Low magnification of a breast biopsy specimen stained for oestrogen receptor protein (ERP) using an immunocytochemical assay (ERICA) shows that most cells are positive (brown). ERICA allows for semiquantitation of ERP. High magnification (inset) reveals that the antibody is localized to the nuclei (brown). (Courtesy of Dr S.L. Khoury, Brigham and Women's Hospital, Boston, MA, USA.)

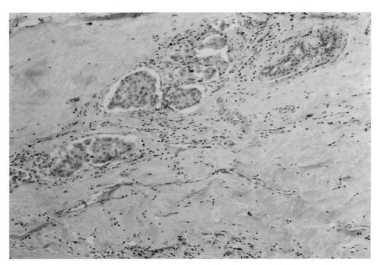

Fig. 3.31 Invasive ductal carcinoma. Photomicroscopic section of a breast biopsy specimen demonstrates an invasive ductal carcinoma in the lymphatic vessels of the breast parenchyma.

Table 3.2 Incidence of histological types of invasive breast cancer

Type	Frequency (%)
Pure tumour groups	68.1
Infiltrating (invasive) ductal	52.6
Medullary	6.2
Lobular invasive	4.9
Mucinous	2.4
Tubular	1.2
Adenocystic	0.4
Papillary	0.3
Carcinosarcoma	0.1
Paget's disease	2.3
Combinations of infiltrating ductal and other types	28.0
Miscellaneous combinations (e.g. tubular + papillary)	1.6

National Surgical Adjuvant Breast Project data; modified from Ref. 22.

highly differentiated tumours that are marked, as their name suggests, by tubule formation. In mucinous (or colloid) carcinomas (see Figure 3.34) nests of neoplastic epithelial cells are surrounded by a mucinous matrix. A few invasive ductal carcinomas exhibit papillary features, hence their designation as papillary carcinomas. Although the above variants may carry a more favourable prognosis than routine infiltrating ductal carcinomas, they are treated similarly, based on stage of disease.

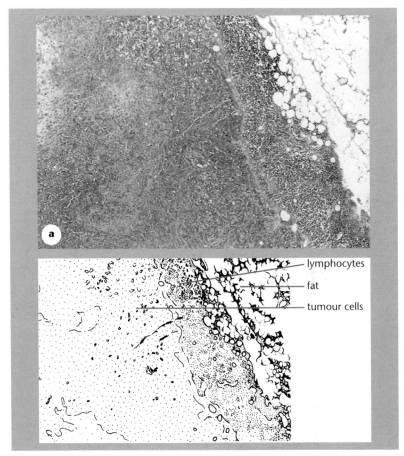

Fig. 3.32 Medullary carcinoma. (a) Low-power photomicrograph of this histological variant of invasive ductal carcinoma demonstrates its characteristic syncytial growth pattern. The tumour has a smooth, well-circumscribed border and exhibits a prominent lymphocytic infiltrate.

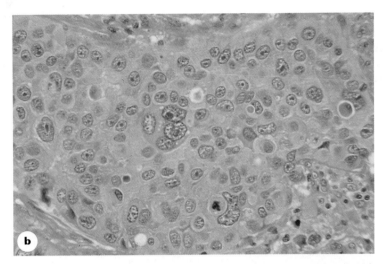

Fig. 3.32 *Continued* (**b**) At higher magnification, the classic pleomorphic cells with bizarre nuclei are evident. This malignancy has better 5- and 10-year survival rates than common ductal carcinoma. (Courtesy of Dr N. Weidner, Brigham and Women's Hospital, Boston, MA, USA.)

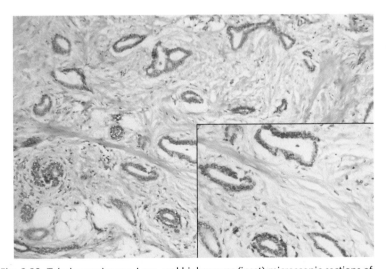

Fig. 3.33 Tubular carcinoma. Low- and high-power (inset) microscopic sections of this histological variant of invasive ductal carcinoma show tubular structures infiltrating the stroma. The lumina of the tubules are lined by a single cell layer of well-differentiated cells. This type of breast cancer has a better prognosis than common infiltrating ductal carcinoma.

About 5–10% of infiltrating cancers arise from the lobules (see Figure 3.35). Histologically, neoplastic cells of these tumours manifest a distinctive 'single-file' pattern. The prognosis and treatment of invasive lobular carcinoma are nearly identical to those of the invasive ductal type. Other unusual malignancies can develop in the breast, including apocrine,

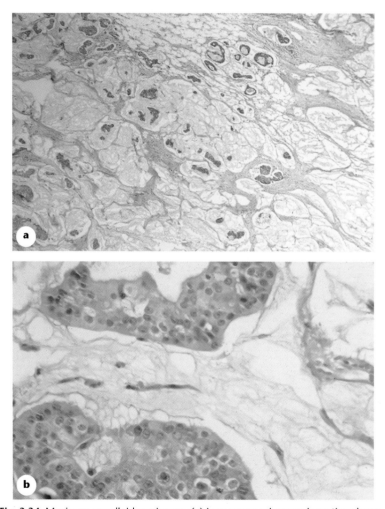

Fig. 3.34 Mucinous or colloid carcinoma. (**a**) Low-power microscopic section shows islands of tumour cells within a sea of mucin. (**b**) Higher magnification demonstrates sharply circumscribed tumour aggregates with characteristic smooth borders and a homogeneous cell population. Pure histological forms of this variant have better prognoses than common ductal carcinoma.

metaplastic, adenoid cystic and squamous cell carcinomas. The cell of origin of the latter three has been difficult to determine. Fibroepithelial malignancies, such as cystosarcoma phylloides, are occasionally found in the breast, arising from the mesenchymal stroma (see Figure 3.36).

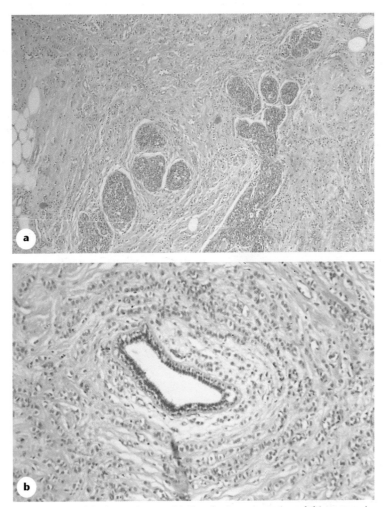

Fig. 3.35 Invasive lobular carcinoma. **(a)** The classic presentation of this tumour is marked by a 'single-file' pattern of uniform malignant cells infiltrating the stroma. The invasive lesion surrounds foci of *in situ* tumour. **(b)** Single-file tumour cells surround an involved duct, producing a target-like pattern.

STAGING OF BREAST CANCER

Staging evaluation consists of a detailed history and physical examination. Particular attention is given to the size, consistency and fixation of the breast mass, skin changes such as erythema, oedema, dimpling and satellite nodules, as well as nipple changes such as retraction, discharge and thickening. The status of axillary and infra- and supraclavicular lymph nodes is also evaluated. Chest and abdominal computed tomograpy (CT) scans and bone scans are performed in patients with node-positive disease or those with localizing symptoms. Head CTs are not routinely done unless patients are experiencing symptoms such as unusual headaches, nausea, cranial nerve deficits and/or gait disturbances.

Classically, staging systems are based on the findings of the clinical examination, in particular on the size of the primary lesion and the extent of metastases to regional lymph nodes (see Figures 3.37 and 3.38). However, in breast cancer, pathological findings are the key to determining an accurate stage (see Table 3.3). In particular, lymph nodes may harbour microscopic metastases (see Figure 3.39). Stage I breast cancers consist of

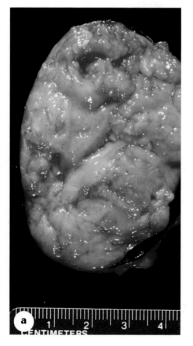

Fig. 3.36 Cystosarcoma phylloides. (**a**) The irregular cut surface of this tumour is marked by clefts that surround glistening grey to yellow islands of tumour intermixed with foci of necrosis (yellow).

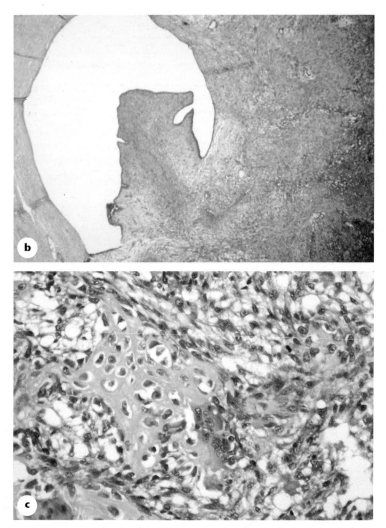

Fig. 3.36 *Continued* (b) Low-magnification study shows the classic leaf-like projection of hypercellular stroma into a benign ductal structure. At high magnification (c), hypercellular areas demonstrate osteosarcomatous differentiation with osteoid (pink) deposition. Scattered 'osteoclast-like' giant cells are also present. Typically, malignant stroma in these tumours appears fibro- or myxoliposarcomatous and less commonly like osteosarcoma, rhabdomysarcoma or chondrosarcoma. (Courtesy of Dr N. Weidner, Brigham and Women's Hospital, Boston, MA, USA.)

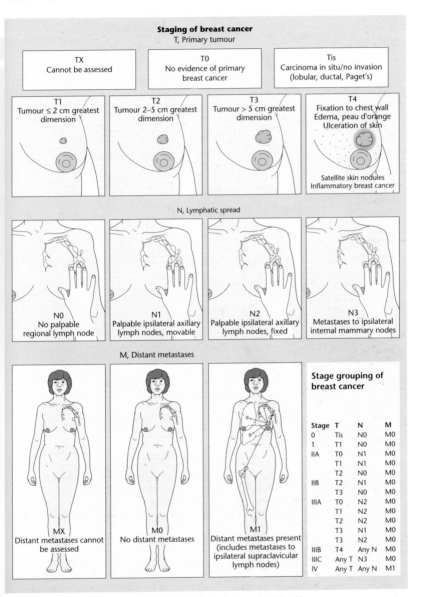

Fig. 3.37 Breast cancer staging based on clinical characteristics.[23]

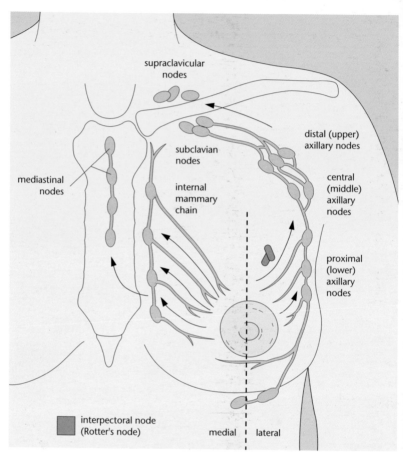

Fig. 3.38 Lymphatic spread of breast cancer. Lymph node metastases are present at the time of diagnosis in up to 60% of cases. In general, lateral lesions in the breast metastasize to the axillary and supraclavicular nodes, whereas medial tumours tend to metastasize to the internal mammary and mediastinal lymph nodes, as well as the supraclavicular nodes. However, lymph node involvement is merely a marker for the probability that the cancer has spread from the breast. A positive finding implies that microdeposits of breast cancer will likely be present in other areas as well.

Table 3.3 Staging criteria for breast cancer. TNM classification.

Primary tumour (T)

TX — Primary tumour cannot be assessed
T0 — No evidence of primary tumour
Tis — Carcinoma *in situ*
- Tis (DCIS) — Intraductal carcinoma *in situ*
- Tis (LCIS) — Lobular carcinoma *in situ*
- Tis (Paget's) — Paget's disease of the nipple with no tumour; tumour-associated Paget's disease is classified according to the size of the primary tumour

T1 — Tumour 2 cm or less in greatest dimension
- T1mic — Microinvasion 0.1 cm or less in greatest dimension
- T1a — Tumour more than 0.1 but not more than 0.5 cm in greatest dimension
- T1b — Tumour more than 0.5 cm but not more than 1 cm in greatest dimension
- T1c — Tumour more than 1 cm but not more than 2 cm in greatest dimension

T2 — Tumour more than 2 cm but not more than 5 cm in greatest dimension
T3 — Tumour more than 5 cm in greatest dimension
T4 — Tumour of any size with direct extension to (a) chest wall or (b) skin, only as described below:
- T4a — Extension to chest wall
- T4b — Oedema (including peau d'orange) or ulceration of the breast skin, or satellite skin nodules confined to the same breast
- T4c — Both (T4a and T4b)
- T4d — Inflammatory carcinoma

Note: Dimpling of the skin, nipple retraction, or any other skin change except those described for T4b and T4d may occur in T1–3 tumours without changing the classification.

Regional lymph nodes (N)

NX — Regional lymph nodes cannot be assessed (e.g. previously removed)
N0 — No regional lymph node metastases
N1 — Metastasis to movable ipsilateral axillary lymph nodes(s)
N2 — Metastasis to ipsilateral axillary lymph node(s) fixed or matted, or in clinically apparent ipsilateral internal mammary nodes in the absence of evident axillary node metastases
- N2a — Metastasis to ipsilateral axillary lymph node(s) fixed to one another (matted) or to other structures
- N2b — Metastasis only in clinically apparent (as detected by imaging studies [excluding lymphoscintigraphy] or by clinical examination or grossly visible pathologically) ipsilateral internal mammary nodes in the absence of evident axillary node metastases

Table 3.3 *Continued* **Staging criteria for breast cancer. TNM classification.**

N3 — Metastasis to ipsilateral infraclavicular lymph node(s) with or without clinically evident axillary lymph nodes, or in clinically apparent ipsilateral internal mammary lymph node(s) and in the presence of clinically evident axillary lymph node metastases, or metastasis in ipsilateral supraclavicular lymph nodes with or without axillary or internal mammary nodal involvement

  • N3a — Metastasis to ipsilateral infraclavicular lymph node(s)
  • N3b — Metastasis to ipsilateral internal mammary lymph node(s) and clinically apparent axillary lymph nodes
  • N3c — Metastasis in ipsilateral supraclavicular lymph nodes with or without axillary or internal mammary nodal involvement

Pathological classification (pN)

Classification is based upon axillary lymph node dissection (ALND) with or without sentinel lymph node dissection (SLND). Classification based solely on SLND without ALND should be designated (sn) [e.g. pN0 (i +) (sn)].

pNX — Regional lymph nodes cannot be assessed (e.g. previously removed, or not removed for pathological study)

pN0 — No regional lymph node metastasis; no additional examination for isolated tumour cells (ITCs, defined as single tumour cells or small clusters not greater than 0.2 mm, usually detected only by immunohistochemical or molecular methods but which may be verified on haematoxylin and eosin (H&E) stains. ITCs do not usually show evidence of malignant activity [e.g. proliferation or stromal reaction])

  • pN0 (i -) — No histological nodal metastases, and negative by immunohistochemistry (IHC)
  • pN0 (i +) — No histological nodal metastases but positive by IHC, with no cluster greater than 0.2 mm in diameter
  • pN0 (mol -) — No histological nodal metastases and negative molecular findings (by reverse transcriptase polymerase chain reaction, RT-PCR)
  • pN0 (mol +) — No histological nodal metastases, but positive molecular findings (by RT-PCR)

pN1 — Metastasis in 1–3 ipsilateral axillary lymph node(s) and/or in internal mammary nodes with microscopic disease detected by SLND but not clinically apparent

  • pN1mi — Micrometastasis (greater than 0.2 mm, none greater than 2.0 mm)
  • pN1a — Metastasis in 1–3 axillary lymph nodes
  • pN1b — Metastasis to internal mammary lymph nodes with microscopic disease detected by SLND but not clinically apparent
  • pN1c — Metastasis in 1–3 ipsilateral axillary lymph node(s) and in internal mammary nodes with microscopic disease detected by SLND but not clinically apparent. If associated with more than three positive axillary nodes, the internal mammary nodes are classified as N3b to reflect increased tumour burden.

Table 3.3 *Continued* **Staging criteria for breast cancer. TNM classification.**

pN2 — Metastasis in 4–9 axillary lymph nodes or in clinically apparent internal mammary lymph nodes in the absence of axillary lymph nodes
- pN2a — Metastases in 4–9 axillary lymph nodes (at least one tumour deposit >2 mm)
- pN2b — Metastasis in clinically apparent internal mammary lymph nodes in the absence of axillary lymph nodes

pN3 — Metastasis in 10 or more axillary lymph nodes, or in infraclavicular lymph nodes, or in clinically apparent ipsilateral internal mammary lymph nodes in the presence of one or more positive axillary nodes; or in more than three axillary lymph nodes with clinically negative microscopic metastasis in internal mammary lymph nodes; or in ipsilateral supraclavicular lymph node(s)
- pN3a — Metastasis in 10 or more axillary lymph nodes (at least one tumour deposit greater than 2.0 mm), or metastasis to the infraclavicular lymph nodes
- pN3b — Metastasis in clinically apparent ipsilateral internal mammary lymph nodes in the presence of one or more positive axillary nodes; or in more than three axillary lymph nodes with microscopic metastasis in internal mammary lymph nodes detected by SLND but not clinically apparent
- pN3c — Metastasis in ipsilateral supraclavicular lymph node(s)

Distant metastasis (M)

MX — Distant metastasis cannot be assessed
M0 — No distant metastasis
M1 — Distant metastasis

Stage groupings

Stage 0 — Tis N0 M0
Stage I — T1 N0 M0 (including T1mic)
Stage IIA — T0 N1 M0; T1 N1 M0 (including T1mic); T2 N0 M0
Stage IIB — T2 N1 M0; T3 N0 M0
Stage IIIA — T0 N2 M0; T1 N2 M0 (including T1mic); T2 N2 M0; T3 N1 M0; T3 N2 M0
Stage IIIB — T4 Any N M0
Stage IIIC — Any T N3 M0
Stage IV — Any T Any N M1

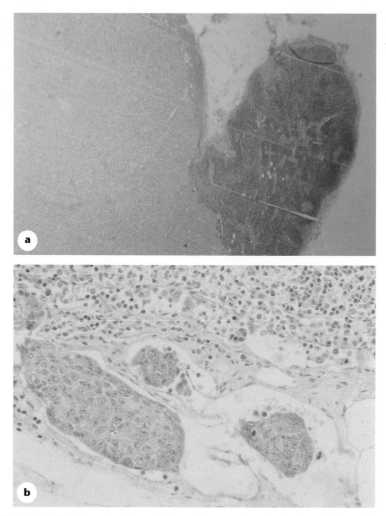

Fig. 3.39 Axillary lymph node metastases. The presence of metastases to the axillary lymph nodes is the single most important prognostic factor in patients with primary breast cancer. **(a)** This lymph node with metastatic breast cancer shows only a small residual area of lymphoid tissue. **(b)** At higher magnification, metastatic deposits can be seen in the subcapsular sinus, a common location for metastases.

small lesions (<2 cm) with no lymph node involvement pathologically; these account for approximately 60% or more of all newly diagnosed breast cancers. Lesions are designated stage II or III by virtue of a larger primary tumour (>2 cm) and/or lymph node involvement. Clinical staging is important in regards to determining if the patient has palpable cervical, supraclavicular, or axillary lymphadenopathy, although these require histological confirmation by fine needle aspiration or biopsy. The diagnosis of inflammatory breast cancer is made on both clinical and pathological grounds (see Figures 3.7 and 3.40–3.44). Patients are considered to have stage IV disease if they have any evidence of distant metastases (see Figure 3.45). Ipsilateral supraclavicular lymphadenopathy is now considered stage IIIC.

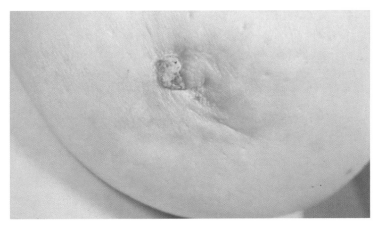

Fig. 3.40 Stage IIIB (T4) breast cancer. A common presentation at this stage is retraction, dimpling and thickening of the skin surrounding the nipple. This clinical finding is designated 'peau d'orange' a name deriving from the pitting and colouration of the skin like orange peel.

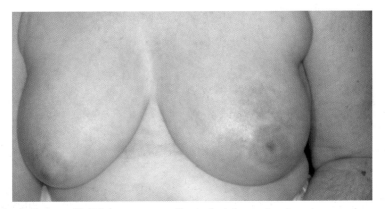

Fig. 3.41 Stage IIB (T4) breast cancer. Classically, inflammatory breast cancer does not present as a discrete mass, but rather as cutaneous erythema with overlying skin warmth, as illustrated in the left breast of this 63-year-old patient.

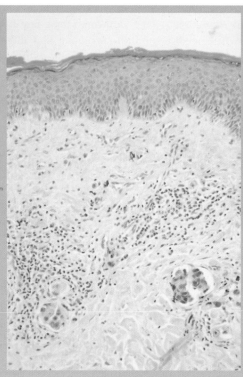

Fig. 3.42 Stage IIIB (T4) breast cancer. The clinical presentation of inflammatory breast cancer is sufficient to make a diagnosis. Yet pathological confirmation of the invasion of dermal lymphatics by malignant cells, as shown in this photomicrograph, can help distinguish this condition from benign mastitis. Note the absence of skin infiltration by inflammatory cells in cancer. The erythema and warmth observed clinically are due to obstruction of dermal lymphatics and subsequent cutaneous lymphoedema.

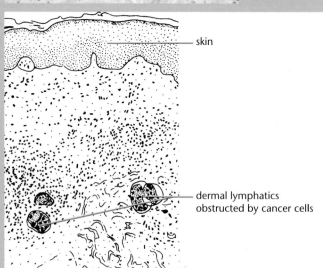

skin

dermal lymphatics obstructed by cancer cells

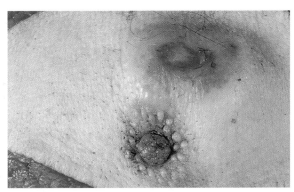

Fig. 3.43 Stage IIIB (T4) breast cancer. Advanced primary carcinomas can present with skin ulceration, as shown in this mastectomy specimen, in the area above the nipple, which is raised and ulcerated by an underlying tumour. Biopsy revealed an adenocarcinoma.

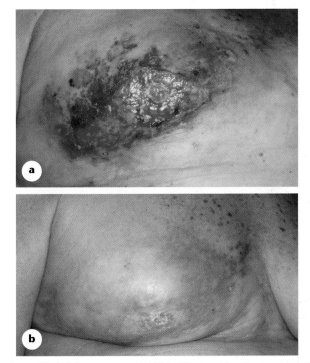

Fig. 3.44 Stage IIIB (T4) breast cancer. (**a**) This 66-year-old patient presented with a locally advanced carcinoma that had ulcerated through the skin, causing substantial morbidity. She was treated effectively with chemotherapy and over 5 months the ulceration decreased as the tumour regressed. (**b**) Ultimately, the skin healed completely.

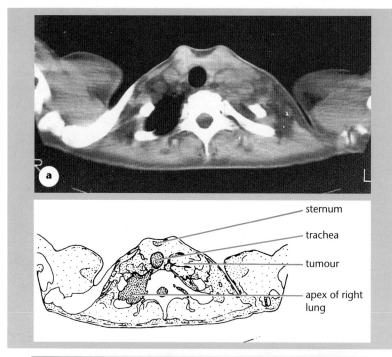

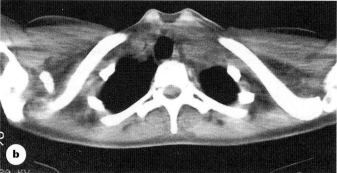

sternum

trachea

tumour

apex of right lung

Fig. 3.45 Supraclavicular/mediastinal metastases. A 35-year-old woman who had undergone lumpectomy and radiotherapy for stage I breast cancer 2 years previously presented with left-sided Horner's syndrome and was found to have a 1 cm hard, fixed nodule in the left supraclavicular fossa. Her chest film demonstrated a soft tissue mass in the left aortopulmonary window. Computed tomography scans of the upper thorax show a soft tissue mass (**a**) filling the left supraclavicular fossa and (**b**) extending interiorly into the left anterior mediastinum. There was no evidence of distant disease. It was of interest that the primary lesion was located in the medial aspect of the left breast and axillary lymph nodes did not contain cancer. The pattern of recurrence shown here probably represents metastasis to the internal mammary lymph node chain.

The heterogeneity of breast cancer is perhaps best illustrated by the wide confidence intervals surrounding the survival curves for each of the staging categories, with considerable overlap between categories. Nonetheless, the presence of metastases to axillary lymph nodes (designated pathological stage II or III) is the single most important prognostic factor in patients with breast cancer. Over 70% of patients with stage I disease are alive 10 years after diagnosis. The survival rates at 5 years for patients with stage II and stage III breast cancer are 50–60% and 30–40%, respectively. Patients with metastatic disease are rarely, if ever, cured and fewer than 10–15% of stage IV patients are alive 5 years after metastases are detected (see Figure 3.46).

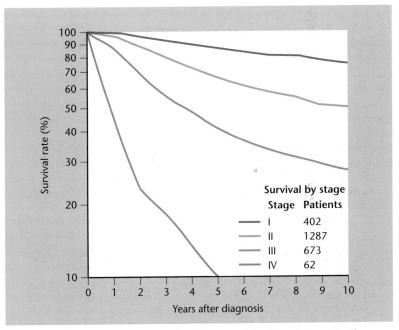

Fig. 3.46 Survival of breast cancer patients by stage at the time of diagnosis. The number of patients diagnosed with each stage is also given.[24]
Of note, the 2002 TNM Staging Classification system was modified as follows:[25]
- Stratification of node staging by the number of involved lymph nodes (0, 1–3, 4–9 and >9)
- Classification of supraclavicular nodes as N3 instead of M1
- Subclassification of nodes based on the extent of involvement and the method of pathological evaluation (H & E versus immunohistochemistry or molecular techniques)

REFERENCES

1. Brinton LA, Schairer C, Hoover RN, Fraumeni JF Jr: Menstrual factors and risk of breast cancer. Cancer Invest 1988; 6(3): 245–254.
2. Negri E, La Vecchia C, Bruzzi P, et al: Risk factors for breast cancer: pooled results from three Italian case-control studies. Am J Epidemiol 1988; 128(6): 1207–1215.
3. Hunter DJ, Spiegelman D, Adami HO, et al: Non-dietary factors as risk factors for breast cancer, and as effect modifiers of the association of fat intake and risk of breast cancer. Cancer Causes Control 1997; 8(1): 49–56.
4. Romieu I, Berlin JA, Colditz G: Oral contraceptives and breast cancer. Review and meta-analysis. Cancer 1990; 66(11): 2253–2263.
5. Collaborative Group on Hormonal Factors in Breast Cancer: Breast cancer and hormonal contraceptives: collaborative reanalysis of individual data on 53 297 women with breast cancer and 100 239 women without breast cancer from 54 epidemiological studies. Lancet 1996; 347(9017): 1713–1727.
6. Trichopoulos D, Hsieh CC, Mac Mahon B, et al: Age at any birth and breast cancer risk. Int J Cancer 1983; 31(6): 701–704.
7. Collaborative Group on Hormonal Factors in Breast Cancer: Breast cancer and breastfeeding: Collaborative reanalysis of individual data from 47 epidemiological studies in 30 countries, including 50302 women with breast cancer and 96973 women without the disease. Lancet 2002; 360(9328): 187–195.
8. Rossouw JE, Anderson GL, Prentice RL, et al: Risks and benefits of estrogen plus progestin in healthy postmenopausal women: principal results from the Women's Health Initiative randomized controlled trial. JAMA 2002; 288(3): 321–333.
9. Ursin G, Longnecker MP, Haile RW, Greenland S: A meta-analysis of body mass index and risk of premenopausal breast cancer. Epidemiology 1995; 6(2): 137–141.
10. van den Brandt PA, Spiegelman D, Yaun SS, et al: Pooled analysis of prospective cohort studies on height, weight, and breast cancer risk. Am J Epidemiol 2000; 152(6): 514–527.
11. Thune I, Brenn T, Lund E, Gaard M: Physical activity and the risk of breast cancer. N Engl J Med 1997; 336(18): 1269–1275.
12. McTiernan A, Kooperberg C, White E, et al: Recreational physical activity and the risk of breast cancer in postmenopausal women: The Women's Health Initiative Cohort Study. JAMA 2003; 290(10): 1331–1336.
13. Key T, Appleby P, Barnes I, et al: Endogenous sex hormones and breast cancer in postmenopausal women: reanalysis of nine prospective studies. J Natl Cancer Inst 2002; 94(8): 606–616.
14. Boyd NF, Lockwood GA, Byng JW, Tritchler DL, Yaffe MJ: Mammographic densities and breast cancer risk. Cancer Epidemiol Biomarkers Prev 1998; 7(12): 1133–1144.
15. Cauley JA, Lucas FL, Kuller LH, et al: Bone mineral density and risk of breast cancer in older women: the study of osteoporotic fractures. Study of Osteoporotic Fractures Research Group [see comments]. JAMA 1996; 276(17): 1404–8.
16. Zhang Y, Kiel DP, Kreger BE, et al: Bone mass and the risk of breast cancer among postmenopausal women. N Engl J Med 1997; 336(9): 611–617.

17. Smith-Warner SA, Spiegelman D, Yaun SS, et al: Alcohol and breast cancer in women: a pooled analysis of cohort studies. JAMA 1998; 279(7): 535–540.
18. Hamajima N, Hirose K, Tajima K, et al: Alcohol, tobacco and breast cancer—collaborative reanalysis of individual data from 53 epidemiological studies, including 58,515 women with breast cancer and 95,067 women without the disease. Br J Cancer 2002; 87(11): 1234–1245.
19. Dupont WD, Page DL: Risk factors for breast cancer in women with proliferative breast disease. N Engl J Med 1985; 312(3): 146–151.
20. Marshall LM, Hunter DJ, Connolly JL, et al: Risk of breast cancer associated with atypical hyperplasia of lobular and ductal types. Cancer Epidemiol Biomarkers Prev 1997; 6(5): 297–301.
21. Collaborative Group on Hormonal Factors in Breast Cancer: Familial breast cancer: collaborative reanalysis of individual data from 52 epidemiological studies including 58,209 women with breast cancer and 101,986 women without the disease. Lancet 2001; 358(9291): 1389–1399.
22. Fisher ER, Gregorio RM, Fisher B, et al: The pathology of invasive breast cancer. A syllabus derived from findings of the National Surgical Adjuvant Breast Project (Protocol No. 4). Cancer 1975; 36: 1.
23. American Joint Committee on Cancer: Manual for staging of cancer, 4th edn. Lippincott, Philadelphia, 1993.
24. Cutler SJ: Classification of extent of disease in breast cancer. Semin Oncol 1974; 1: 91.
25. Greene FL, Page DL, Fleming ID, et al: AJCC cancer staging manual, 6th edn. Springer-Verlag, New York, 2002.

FURTHER READING

Berg JW, Hutter RVP: Breast cancer, histology of cancer. Incidence and prognosis: SEER population-based data, 1973–1987. Cancer 1995; 75: 257–269.

Early Breast Cancer Trialists' Collaborative Group T: Systemic treatment of early breast cancer by hormonal, cytotoxic, or immune therapy: 133 randomized trials involving 31,000 recurrences and 24,000 deaths among 75,000 women. Lancet 1992; 339: 1–15, 71–85.

Fisher B, Costantino J, Redmond C, et al: Lumpectomy compared with lumpectomy and radiation therapy for the treatment of intraductal breast cancer. N Engl J Med 1993; 328: 1581–1586.

Fisher B, Costantino J, Redmond C, et al: Endometrial cancer in tamoxifen-treated breast cancer patients: Findings from the National Surgical Adjuvant Breast and Bowel Project (NSAPBP). J Natl Cancer Inst 1994; 86: 527–537.

Gabriel S, O'Fallon W, Kurland L, et al: Risk of connective-tissue disease and other disorders after breast implantation. N Engl J Med 1994; 330: 1697–1702.

Greenlee, RT, Murray T, Bolden S, Wingo PA: Cancer statistics, 2000. CA Cancer J Clin 2000; 50(1): 7–33.

Harris J, Hellman S, Henderson IC, et al: Breast diseases, 2nd edn. Lippincott, Philadelphia, 1990.

Harris JR, Lippman ME, Veronesi U, Willett W: Breast cancer. Part 1. N Engl J Med 1992; 327: 319–328.

Hayes DF, ed: Atlas of breast cancer. Mosby Europe, London, 1993.

Hayes DF: Tumor markers for breast cancer. Ann Oncol 1993; 4: 807–819.

Hayes DF, Henderson, IC, Shapiro, CL: Treatment of metastatic breast cancer: present and future prospect. Semin Oncol 1995; 22: 5–21.

Kelsey JL, Berkowitz GS: Breast cancer epidemiology. Cancer Res 1988; 48: 5615–5623.

Lumb G, Mackenzie DH: The incidence of metastases in adrenal glands and ovaries removed for cancer of the breast. Cancer 1959; 12: 521–526.

McGuire WL, Clark GM: Prognostic factors and treatment decisions in axillary node-negative breast cancer. N Engl J Med 1992; 326: 1756–1761.

Merkel DE, Osborne CK: Prognostic factors in breast cancer. Hematol Oncol Clin North Am 1989; 3: 641–652.

Miki Y, Shattuck-Eldens D, Futreal PA, et al: Isolation of BRCA1, the 17q-linked breast and ovarian cancer susceptibility gene. Science 1994; 266: 61–71.

Schnitt SJ, Sadowsky NL, Connolly JL, et al: Ductal carcinoma in situ (intraductal carcinoma) of the breast. N Engl J Med 1988; 318: 898–903.

Shapiro CL, Henderson IC: New directions in breast cancer. Saunders, Philadelphia, 1994.

Smart C, Hendrick RE, Rutledge J, et al: Benefit of mammography screening in women aged 40–49 years. Cancer 1995; 75: 1619–1626.

Stomper PC, Gelman RS: Mammography in symptomatic and asymptomatic patients. Hematol Oncol Clin North Am 1989; 3: 611–640.

Vasconez LO, LeJour H, Gamboa-Bobadilla M: Atlas of breast reconstruction. Gower, New York, 1991.

Veronesi U, Paganelli G, Galimberti V, et al: Sentinel-node biopsy to avoid axillary dissection in breast cancer with clinically negative lymph nodes. Lancet 1997; 349: 1864–1867.

FIGURE CREDITS

The following books published by Gower Medical Publishing are gratefully acknowledged as sources of figures in the present chapter.

Hayes DF, ed: Atlas of Breast Cancer. Mosby Europe, London, 1993.

Fig 3.44: Fletcher CDM, McKee PH: An Atlas of Gross Pathology. Edward Arnold/Gower Medical Publishing, London, 1987, p. 47.

Breast cancer therapy

4

Wendy Y. Chen

PRIMARY TREATMENT

In the late 19th century, the technique of mastectomy was pioneered by Halsted and found to improve local control of breast cancer. For the next 50–75 years, the concept that breast cancer spread in an orderly fashion from the primary lesion to regional lymph nodes and then to distant organs dominated the treatment of early disease (see Figures 4.1 and 4.2). During this time, radical mastectomy (the complete removal of the breast, pectoral muscles and axillary contents) was the treatment of choice. Subsequent studies have demonstrated that patients treated with less aggressive (modified radical) mastectomies have the same survival as those treated with radical mastectomies. In the last 15 years, breast-conserving therapy, in which the initial mass is removed by 'lumpectomy' or 'quadrantectomy', followed by primary radiation to the remainder of the breast, has been shown to produce survival rates similar to those seen with treatment by mastectomy. In most cases less aggressive, breast-conserving local therapy provides excellent cosmetic results (see Figures 4.3 and 4.4).

There are also new advances in exploring the axilla for the determination of lymph node involvement. A sentinel axillary lymph node is the first area to receive lymph flow and is usually the first to harbour a metastasis from the breast cancer. In selected patients a sentinel node biopsy serves as a means of avoiding a complete axillary dissection. In experienced hands a sentinel node biopsy is the preferred manner to assess disease in the axilla. To localize the sentinel node, surgeons inject one or two markers, blue dye or as technetium sulphur colloid-technetium-99m, around the tumour or biopsy cavity. The markers are taken up into the lymphatic channels surrounding the tumour site and travel to the nodal basin. In some situations lymphoscintigraphy is performed after the injection to map out the lymphatic drainage pattern. A positive sentinel node requires a full axillary dissection (see Figure 4.5). If the sentinel node biopsy is negative a full axillary dissection can be spared, eliminating the known potential complications of a dissection such as lymphoedema (see Figure 4.6).

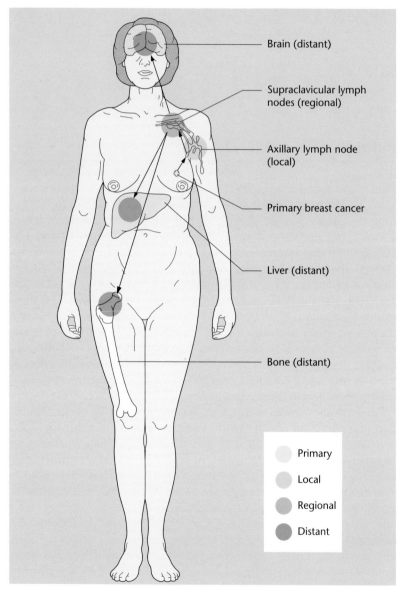

Brain (distant)

Supraclavicular lymph nodes (regional)

Axillary lymph node (local)

Primary breast cancer

Liver (distant)

Bone (distant)

Primary

Local

Regional

Distant

Fig. 4.1 Halsted theory of breast cancer spread. This theory suggests that breast cancer originates in the breast, eventually spreads to local skin and/or lymph nodes and then ultimately affects distant organs. This theory maintains that local/regional lymph nodes serve as 'barriers' to the spread of metastatic breast cancer. The implication of this theory is that more intensive local therapy should lead to an increased rate of cures.

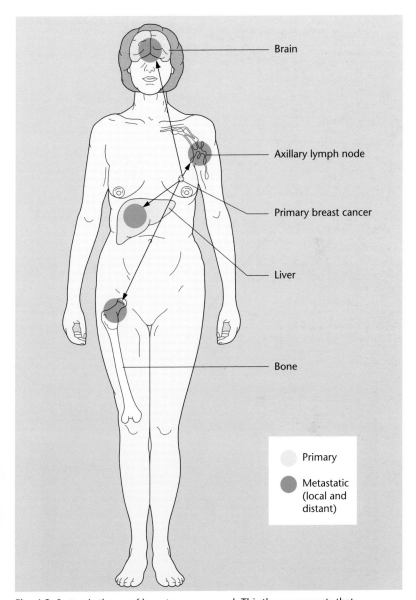

Fig. 4.2 Systemic theory of breast cancer spread. This theory suggests that breast cancer becomes metastatic very early in its course, once invasion through the basement membrane of the duct or lobule has occurred. It maintains that local therapy will have few if any long-term effects on survival, since the disease is already systemic at the time of diagnosis.

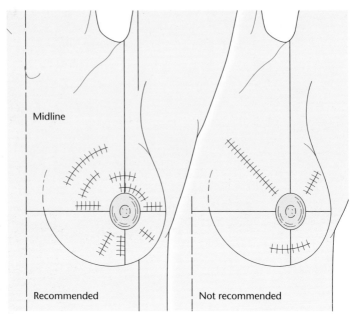

Fig. 4.3 Cosmesis is best maintained using circular incisions in the upper half of the breast and radial incisions in the lower half of the breast.

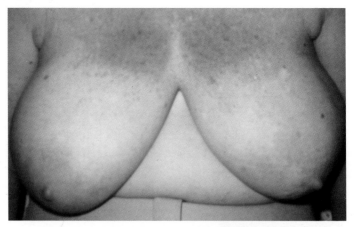

Fig. 4.4 The cosmetic results of conservative therapy are usually quite satisfactory. This 70-year-old patient had a stage I carcinoma of the left breast that was treated by excisional biopsy and primary irradiation. Although there is some asymmetry of the breast, as well as, on close inspection, some modest skin thickening and retraction due to the therapy, it is very difficult to determine which breast was treated.

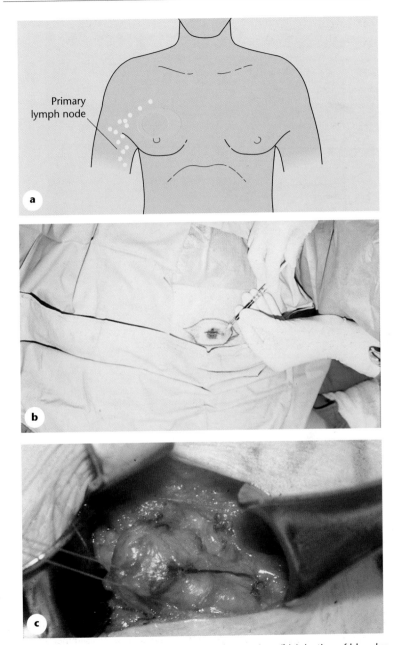

Fig. 4.5 Sentinel node biopsy. (**a**) Axillary lymph mapping. (**b**) Injection of blue dye in the tumour cavity. (**c**) Identification of the sentinel node (follow blue line).

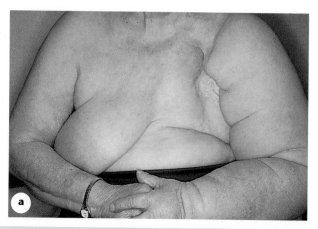

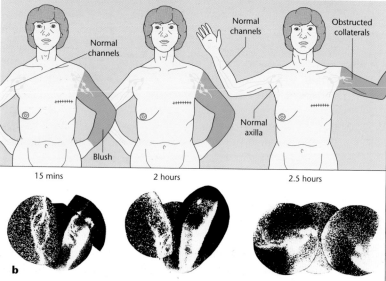

Fig. 4.6 (a) A 64-year-old patient with significant arm oedema after a radical mastectomy, full axillary dissection and postoperative chest wall and axillary radiotherapy. The patient's left arm is immensely swollen in contrast to her unaffected, normal right arm. After subcutaneous injection of radionuclide into the dorsum of each hand, scintigrams were obtained (b). In the anterior views at 15 minutes and 2 hours, flow can easily be seen in normal channels in the right arm. However, only a 'blush' can be seen in the left arm because the normal lymph channels are occluded and the radionuclide is present only in small collateral channels that do not communicate with distal vessels. In the view of the thorax at 2.5 hours, flow can be seen on the right side in normal channels leading to axillary lymph nodes. In contrast, radionuclide has accumulated in the lower arm and is absent in the left axilla.

The completion of breast conservation therapy involves radiation therapy. The whole breast is treated using a pair of tangentially directed fields. The fields are designed to skim along the chest wall and thus irradiate the smallest amount of underlying lung. At the conclusion of the whole breast treatment a boost dose is often given to the tumour bed. Such conservative therapy, however, is not appropriate for all patients. Contraindications include multicentric disease, diffuse malignant microcalcifications and previous breast radiation therapy. For those who require or prefer mastectomies, remarkable advances have been made in recent years in reconstructive surgery (see Figures 4.7–4.11).

ADJUVANT THERAPY

Adjuvant therapy refers to systemic treatment given after surgical removal of the breast tumour. The rationale for adjuvant therapy for breast cancer is that occult micrometastatic disease may exist even after a breast tumour has been completely removed. If untreated, the micrometastatic disease could potentially lead to the development of distant recurrences. Adjuvant therapy can consist of hormonal therapy, chemotherapy or biological therapies, such as trastuzumab. Later in this chapter, factors such as oestrogen/progesterone and Her2neu status, which help drive treatment choices, will be discussed. First, methods to estimate an individual's risk of recurrence will be introduced.

ESTIMATING RECURRENCE RISK

Decision making for adjuvant therapy for breast cancer is strongly driven by estimates of a person's risk of recurrence. Although the relative benefits of chemotherapy and hormonal therapy appear similar for both low- and high-risk women, the absolute additional benefits associated with adjuvant therapy will differ by the underlying risk of recurrence.

Adjuvant! Online
The most widely used statistical model in the US is Adjuvant! Online (available free of charge at www.adjuvantonline.com). Developed by Dr Peter Ravdin and colleagues, Adjvuant! Online utilizes data from SEER (Surveillance, Epidemiology, and End Results) and the EBCTTG (Early Breast Cancer Trialists Collaborative Group) overview to estimate disease-free and overall survival with various treatment options, also taking into account death from non-breast cancer causes.[1] Required data are:

age at diagnosis, comorbidity (perfect health, minor, average for age, major – three categories), estrogen receptor (ER) status, tumour grade, tumour size (0.1–1.0, 1.1–2.0, 2.1–3.0, 3.1–5.0, >5.0 cm) and number of positive nodes (0, 1–3, 4–9, >9). The program then calculates 10-year

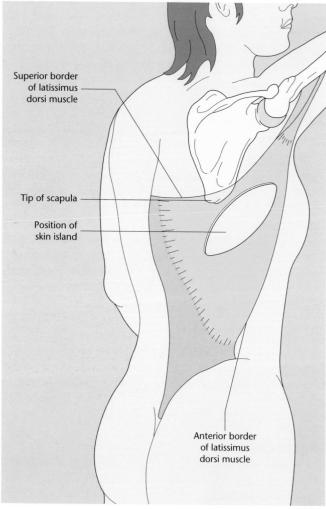

Superior border of latissimus dorsi muscle

Tip of scapula

Position of skin island

Anterior border of latissimus dorsi muscle

Fig. 4.7 Breast reconstructive surgery. The latissimus dorsi myocutaneous flap is based on the thoracodorsal artery and vein. This flap is rotated from the back and becomes the breast mound.[167] Alternatively, a transverse rectus abdominis muscle (TRAM) flap can be used, which is advantageous in large-breasted women when additional tissue coverage is needed.

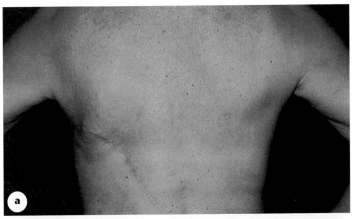

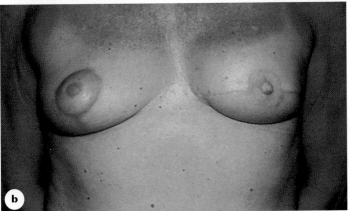

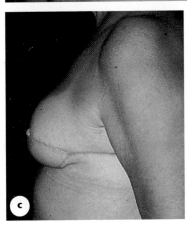

Fig. 4.8 (a) The resultant scar from harvesting a latissimus flap. (b,c) The resulting cosmetic effect after reconstruction with a latissimus flap.

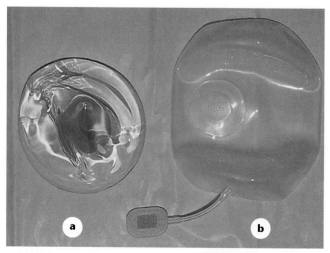

Fig. 4.9 Silicone implant (a) and tissue expander inflated with saline (b).

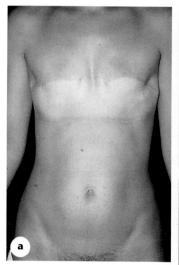

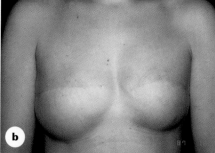

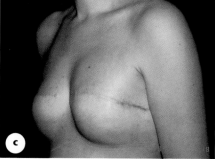

Fig. 4.10 (a) A patient with bilateral mastectomies. (b,c) Frontal and side views of the same patient after bilateral silicone implants.

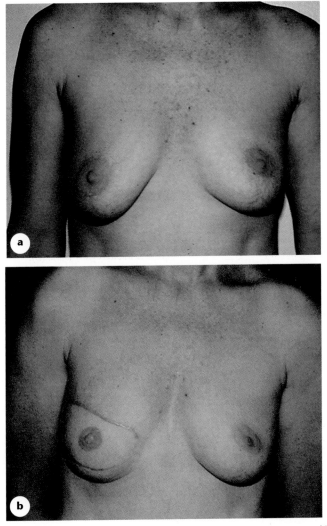

Fig. 4.11 (a) Before mastectomy. (b) The same patient after mastectomy and TRAM (see Figure 4.7) flap reconstruction.

risks of recurrence and overall mortality. Overall mortality takes into account deaths from both breast cancer and other causes. Estimates for benefits of various hormonal therapy (tamoxifen for 5 years, aromatase inhibitor for 5 years, sequential therapy with tamoxifen followed by an aromatase inhibitor, ovarian ablation, and tamoxifen + ovarian ablation) and chemotherapy (cyclophosphamide, methotrexate and 5FU (CMF) and various anthracycline- and taxane-containing regimens) regimens are calculated. From its initial model, other models incorporating results from OncotypeDX testing and estimating benefit for letrozole after 5 years of tamoxifen for ER-positive cancers have been developed. Currently, Her2neu is not used as part of the prognostic model and therefore none of the chemotherapy estimates account for the effects of trastuzumab. The estimates from Advjuant! Online have been validated in a separate population-based dataset.[2]

OncotypeDX testing

Another way to estimate recurrence risk is utilizing gene expression data from the tumour. Although multiple investigators have published on this topic, OncotypeDX has several advantages:

1. it is commercially available
2. it utilized large randomized controlled trials for model development
3. it can be performed on formalin-fixed, paraffin-embedded tissue, an important practical consideration since that represents the most common storage form for tumours obtained during routine breast cancer surgery.

OncotypeDX is a reverse transcriptase-polymerase chain reaction-based assay of 16 cancer and five reference genes (see Table 4.1). The initial dataset for model building drew upon three clinical trials to estimate 10-year risks of distant recurrence. The assay was then validated using subjects from NSABP-14, a randomized trial of tamoxifen compared with placebo in ER-positive, node-negative breast cancer (see Figure 4.12).[3] The results have been validated in both the tamoxifen and placebo arms of the National Surgical Adjuvant Breast Project NSABP-14 and NSABP-20, although a smaller study from MD Anderson showed lesser degrees of concordance.[4]

In addition, the authors have published data estimating the amount of benefit from adjuvant chemotherapy.[5] Patients with a high recurrence score (≥ 31) derived a large benefit from chemotherapy (relative risk (RR) 0.26, 95%) CI 0.13–0.53, correlating with an absolute difference of 27.6% in 10-year distant recurrence rates), whereas those with a low recurrence score (<18) did not derive a benefit (RR 1.31, 95% CI

0.46–3.78, p for interaction =0.038). However, it should be noted that OncotypeDX has not been used yet prospectively to determine the benefit of adjuvant chemotherapy. Trials to validate gene-expression-based assays (TAILORx and MINDACCT) are currently underway in North America and Europe.[6] In addition, OncotypeDX can only be used in women with ER-positive, node-negative breast cancer, since it has not been validated in node-positive or ER-negative populations.

GUIDELINES FOR ADJUVANT TREATMENT

The two large groups that publish comprehensive guidelines for the adjuvant treatment of breast cancer are National Comprehensive Cancer Network (NCCN) and the International Expert Consensus Panel (St. Gallen). NCCN tends to reflect practice patterns in the US whereas St. Gallen reflects European patterns.

Table 4.1 The 21 genes used for OncotypeDX assay[3]

- *GSTM1*
- *CD68*
- *BAG1*
- **Proliferation**
    Ki67
    STK15
    Survivin
    CCNB1 (cyclin B1)
    MYBL2
- **Invasion**
    MMP11 (stromolysin 3)
    CTSL2 (capthepsin L2)
- **HER2**
    GRB7
    HER2
- **Oestrogen**
    ER (oestrogen receptor)
    PGR (progesterone receptor)
    BCL2
    SCUBE2
- **Reference**
    ACTB (beta-actin)
    GAPDH
    RPLPO
    GUS
    TFRC

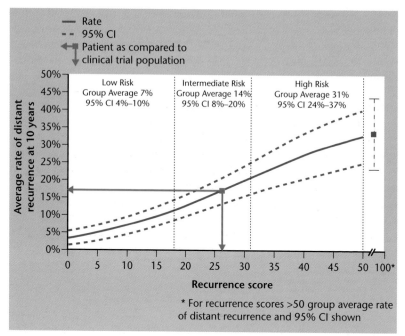

Fig. 4.12 Hypothetical example of the OncotypeDX results for a woman with a recurrence score of 26 which correlate with an average rate of distant recurrence at 10 years of 17% (95% confidence interval 13–21%). Adapted from Paik S, Shak S, Tang G, et al: A multigene assay to predict recurrence of tamoxifen-treated, node-negative breast cancer. N Engl J Med 2004; 351: 2817–2826.

NCCN guidelines

NCCN guidelines are available on the web at www.nccn.org and are updated annually. Treatment guidelines are based upon tumour size, node status (positive vs. negative), ER/PR (progesterone receptor), Her2neu and menopausal status (for hormonal therapy). In addition, 'unfavourable features' (high histological grade, Her2neu status, presence of angiolymphatic invasion) are considered for node-negative patients with tumours ≤1 cm. Recommendations regarding surgery and radiation therapy are also included.

Based upon NCCN guidelines, all women with ER-positive cancers will be recommended adjuvant hormonal therapy. Chemotherapy is recommended for all node-positive women and node-negative women with tumours >1 cm regardless of ER status (with the exception of certain favourable histologies such as tubular carcinomas), although the strength of the recommendation varies depending upon the specific tumour characteristics. For tumours measuring 0.6–1.0 cm, chemotherapy can be considered for those with adverse features, such as high histological grade or presence of lymphatic vascular invasion. Trastuzumab is recommended for all Her2neu positive tumours that are node positive or high-risk node negative.

International Consensus Panel (St. Gallen)

In contrast, the St. Gallen group utilized slightly different criteria. Women are divided into low-, medium- or high-risk categories based upon factors including tumour size (≤ or >2 cm), histological grade (1 vs. 2–3), lymphatic vascular invasion, Her2neu status, age (< or ≥35 years) and nodal status (negative, 1–3 positive nodes, four or more positive nodes) (see Table 4.2). Hormone responsiveness is no longer used as part of risk categorization, but is used to drive treatment recommendations (see Table 4.3). Decisions for chemotherapy are more strongly driven by hormone receptor status than with the NCCN guidelines. Specific differences are discussed in the following section.

Differences between NCCN and St. Gallen criteria

In general, the NCCN guidelines are more likely to recommend adjuvant chemotherapy for node-negative women compared with St. Gallen. For example, the NCCN recommends adjuvant chemotherapy for all women with tumours >1 cm, regardless of hormone receptor, Her2neu or nodal status. The St. Gallen criteria only recommend chemotherapy for women considered intermediate or high risk. The NCCN criteria also recommend

Table 4.2 St. Gallen criteria[165]		
Risk categories	**Nodal status**	**Necessary features**
Low risk	Node negative	Tumour ≤2 cm AND Grade 1 AND absence of peritumoral vessel invasion AND Her2neu negative AND age ≥35 years
Intermediate risk	Node negative	Tumour >2 cm OR grade 2–3 OR presence of peritumoral vessel invasion OR Her2neu positive OR age <35 years
	1–3 positive nodes	Her2neu negative
High risk	1–3 positive nodes	Her2neu positive
	4 or more positive nodes	Any histology or Her2neu status

Table 4.3 St. Gallen guidelines[165]

Risk category	Endocrine responsive	Endocrine response uncertain	Endocrine non-responsive
Low risk	Endocrine therapy OR Nil	Endocrine therapy OR Nil	Not applicable
Intermediate risk	Endocrine therapy only OR Chemotherapy + endocrine therapy (sequential or concurrent)	Chemotherapy + endocrine therapy	Chemotherapy
High risk	Chemotherapy + endocrine therapy (sequential or concurrent)	Chemotherapy + endocrine therapy	Chemotherapy

adjuvant trastuzumab for all women with node-positive, Her2neu-positive breast cancer. The 2005 St. Gallen panel was convened before publication of the adjuvant trastuzumab data, so did not incorporate any recommendations regarding trastuzumab.

HORMONAL THERAPY

Since Dr George Beatson's observations over 100 years ago that metastatic breast cancer would regress after an oophorectomy, it has been recognized that many breast cancers are strongly influenced by hormonal factors. In the 1950s, ovarian suppression was used both for the treatment of metastatic disease and as adjuvant therapy. Tumours that express either oestrogen and/or progesterone receptors are considered to be hormonally sensitive and may respond to adjuvant hormonal therapy.

Tamoxifen

Tamoxifen, a selective oestrogen receptor modulator (SERM) has both oestrogen antagonist and agonist effects. Its antagonist effect at the level of the oestrogen receptor explains its therapeutic benefit. Its agonist effects give rise to both favourable (e.g. improvement of bone density) and unfavourable (e.g. increased risk of endometrial cancer) side effects. Tamoxifen has been shown to be effective as adjuvant breast cancer treatment both for pre- and postmenopausal women. In this section, we will review the data on the use of tamoxifen in the adjuvant setting.

The most comprehensive examination of tamoxifen as adjuvant therapy has been conducted by the EBCTCG .[7] In the most recent 2005 publication, the overview pooled centrally collected data from randomized controlled trials conducted worldwide that had started by 1995 to calculate 10- and 15-year outcomes. As expected, tamoxifen only benefited women with ER-positive disease, defined as ≥10 fmol/mg cytosol protein by biochemical assay or any immunhistochemical staining (see Table 4.4). All numbers quoted below are for women with ER-positive cancers. Adjuvant tamoxifen was associated with a decrease in breast cancer recurrence and death rates, most strongly for 5 years of use. For women who did not receive chemotherapy but completed 5 years of tamoxifen, annual recurrence rates and death rates were decreased by 41% (SE 0.03) and 34% (SE 0.03), respectively. This translates to an absolute difference at 15 years for breast cancer recurrence and death of 11.8% (45% control vs. 33.2% tamoxifen arms) and 9.2% (34.8% control vs. 25.6% tamoxifen arms), respectively. It should also be noted that the benefits of tamoxifen persisted despite discontinuation after 5 years of use, and actually increased over time. The benefit of tamoxifen at 15 years was greater than that at 5 years. Included in the estimates of recurrence rates were a decreased risk of contralateral breast cancer (RR 0.61, 95% CI 0.50–0.73).

Dose and duration
The standard dose of tamoxifen is 20 mg daily (or 10 mg bid). There does not appear to be any benefit to higher doses of tamoxifen. Five years of

Table 4.4 Adjuvant tamoxifen, Oxford overview[7]		
	Rate ratio comparing tamoxifen with control (SE)	
	Breast cancer recurrence	Breast cancer mortality
1–2 years of tamoxifen		
ER poor	0.89 (0.04)	0.91 (0.04)
ER positive	0.74 (0.02)	0.82 (0.03)
5 years of tamoxifen		
ER poor	1.04 (0.07)	1.04 (0.08)
ER positive	0.59 (0.03)	0.66 (0.04)
ER, oestrogen receptor.		

tamoxifen was superior to 1–2 years of tamoxifen. Several trials have compared 10 years with 5 years of tamoxifen, but all still have a relatively small number of recurrences. For women with lymph node-negative breast cancer there does not seem to be any additional benefit to continuing tamoxifen beyond 5 years. There may even be an adverse effect based upon NSABP B-14[8] and the Scottish Adjuvant Tamoxifen trial,[9] although these differences were not statistically significant. However, an Eastern Cooperative Oncology Group trial in node-positive women demonstrated a statistically significant improvement in time to relapse, but not in overall survival, for women who continued tamoxifen for more than 5 years.[10] However, given the data in node-negative patients, the current recommendation is discontinuation of tamoxifen after 5 years of treatment for women who are not candidates for treatment with an aromatase inhibitor.

Sequencing of tamoxifen with chemotherapy

The EBCTCG overview did not comment on sequencing of tamoxifen (concurrent vs. sequential) with regard to chemotherapy administration since no large randomized trials directly addressed this question during the study period. The sequencing issue arose because of concern that the cytostatic effect of tamoxifen might interfere with the efficacy of cytotoxic chemotherapy. However, several randomized trials have suggested a benefit to sequential treatment with chemotherapy followed by tamoxifen, although neither were statistically significant using a two-sided p-value of 0.05.[11,12]

Sequencing of tamoxifen with radiation

Several trials have evaluated the sequencing of radiotherapy and tamoxifen. Again, preclinical data suggested that breast cancer cells may have reduced radiosensitivity when treated with tamoxifen.[13,14] Although no randomized trial has directly addressed this question, several large retrospective studies have recently evaluated this issue. All three studies showed no significant difference in rates of ipsilateral tumour recurrence and disease-free or overall survival.[15–17] Therefore, there does not appear to be a strong effect from sequencing of tamoxifen and radiation therapy, but a large randomized trial would be necessary to definitively answer this question.

Other factors and tamoxifen effect

For women with ER-positive disease, chemotherapy did not appear to modify the effect of tamoxifen, or the converse. Tamoxifen and chemotherapy was superior to chemotherapy alone. The relative effects of tamoxifen did not vary by age at diagnosis, nodal status or menopausal status.

Side effects

Because of its antagonist and agonist properties, tamoxifen is associated with effects outside those on breast cancer recurrence. Most of these data have been drawn from the prevention trials in which women without a history of breast cancer were randomized either to tamoxifen or placebo, a better population to evaluate than breast cancer patients who may be at an increased risk of secondary cancers or have a hypercoagulable state. One of the largest prevention trials was NSABP P-1, which randomized 13,388 women without a personal history of invasive breast cancer but with a higher risk of developing breast cancer to either tamoxifen or placebo.[18] There was a statistically significant decrease in osteoporotic fractures (RR 0.68, 95% CI 0.51–0.92) for tamoxifen. However, tamoxifen was also associated with a statistically significant increased risk of invasive endometrial cancer (RR 3.28, 95% CI 1.87–6.03) and pulmonary embolus (RR 2.15, 95% CI 1.08–4.51), mainly in women 50 years of age or older, and also an increased rate of cataracts and cataract surgery. There was also a non-statistically significant increase in risk of stroke (RR 1.42, 95% CI 0.97–2.08) and deep venous thrombosis with tamoxifen (RR 1.44, 95% CI 0.91–2.30). Tamoxifen did not effect the development of ischaemic heart disease. An overview of five large randomized prevention trials (NSABP P-1, Royal Marsden, Italian prevention study, IBIS-1, MORE) showed similar relative risks.[19] Short-term side effects are common and include vaginal discharge and menopausal symptoms, such as hot flashes and vaginal dryness.

Aromatase inhibitors

For postmenopausal women, aromatase inhibitors (AI) are frequently used in addition to or instead of tamoxifen. This class of drugs, which includes anastrozole, letrozole and exemestane, blocks the action of aromatase, the enzyme responsible for the conversion of androgenic precursors to oestrogens. Anastrozole and letrozole are non-steroidal reversible AI, whereas exemestane is a steroidal irreversible AI. In postmenopausal women, AI cause a marked diminution in circulating oestrogen levels. AI are not used in premenopausal women because the decrease in oestrogen level can feed back on the pituitary/hypothalamus causing gonadotropin secretion and ovarian stimulation. The AI trials were not included in the most recent EBCTCG overview, but at least five trials have shown similar results using AI as adjuvant hormonal therapy, either up front or sequentially with tamoxifen. The first study published was ATAC (Anastrozole, Tamoxifen, Alone or in Combination) in which postmenopausal women with ER-positive/unknown cancers were randomized to anastrozole alone at 1 mg daily (N = 3125), tamoxifen alone at 20 mg daily (N = 3116) or the combination (N = 3125).[20,21] At the time of a preplanned interim analysis with median follow-up of 33 months, the combination arm was closed since results for the combination arm were similar to the tamoxifen-alone arm. All results reported below are for the comparison of anastrozole with tamoxifen (see Figure 4.13). In the most recent update with a median follow-up of 68 months, compared with tamoxifen alone, anastrozole was associated with a significant improvement in disease-free survival (RR 0.87, 95% CI 0.78–0.97, p=0.01) and reduction of distant metastases (RR 0.86, 95% CI 0.74–0.99,

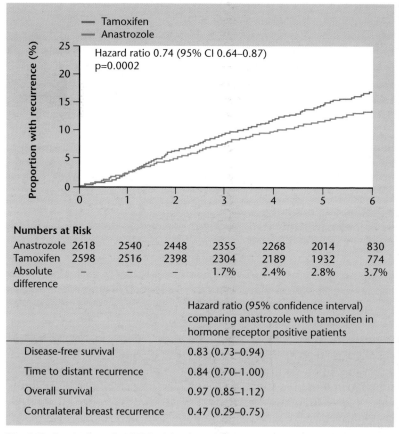

Fig. 4.13 Results from the ATAC trial. Adapted from Howell A, Cuzick J, et al: Results of the ATAC (Arimidex, Tamoxifen, Alone or in Combination) trial after completion of 5 years' adjuvant treatment for breast cancer. Lancet 2005; 365(9453): 60–62.

p=0.04) and contralateral breast cancers (RR 0.58, 95% CI 0.38–0.88, p=0.01). There was no difference in overall survival (RR 0.97, 95% CI 0.85–1.12, p=0.7). Similar early results were seen in the BIG 1-98 trial, which thus far has only reported on the upfront comparison of letrozole to tamoxifen.[22]

Several other randomized trials have also investigated the sequential use of AI after initial treatment with tamoxifen. The first published and largest of these studies was the MA-17 trial, which randomized 5,124 postmenopausal women with ER- and/or PR- positive cancers to letrozole 2.5 mg daily or placebo after completion of 5 years of tamoxifen. The study was unblinded with a median follow-up of 2.4 years when there was a statistically significant improvement in disease-free survival favouring the letrozole arm at the time of a preplanned interim analysis.[23] An updated analysis with median follow up of 2.5 years showed no difference in overall survival between the two arms (RR 0.82, 95% CI 0.57–1.19, p=0.3 comparing letrozole with tamoxifen). However, there was a statistically significant improvement in overall survival among the subgroup of lymph node-positive patients (RR 0.61, 95% CI 0.38–0.98, p=0.04).[24] In addition, four other randomized trials have investigated an AI after 2–3 years of tamoxifen. All showed similar results with an improvement in disease-free survival, but not overall survival favouring the AI.[25–27]

Hot flashes, vaginal symptoms and thromboembolic events are less common with AI compared with tamoxifen. However, the AI are associated with a higher incidence of arthralgias and bone density loss leading to an increased risk of fractures and osteoporosis.[20–22] The optimal duration of AI use is still not known.

Ovarian ablation/suppression

For premenopausal women, ovarian ablation or suppression can also be considered as an additional adjuvant option. Ovarian ablation can be achieved either through surgery or ovarian irradiation; ovarian suppression through the use of luteinizing hormone-releasing hormone (LHRH) agonists. There does not seem to be a difference in outcome depending upon the type of ovarian ablation/suppression. However, it should be noted that the effects of LHRH agonists on ovarian function are reversible after discontinuation of the drug, as opposed to the permanent effects of surgery or radiation.

Again, the most comprehensive data on this topic have been compiled by the EBCTCG, which pooled data on almost 8,000 women younger than 50 years of age.[7] The data reported below pertain only to women with ER-positive or ER-unknown cancers. Compared with no treatment, ovarian ablation or suppression was associated with an improvement in 15-year rates for recurrence (difference = 4.3%, SE 1.9) and breast cancer mortality (difference 3.2%, SE 2.0). Compared indirectly with studies of tamoxifen effects, the effects of ovarian suppression/ablation appear to be of smaller magnitude. The optimal duration of ovarian suppression is also not known. Studies have evaluated lengths from 2 to 5 years (see Table 4.5).

Ovarian ablation/suppression compared with chemotherapy alone
Although the EBCTCG overview did not directly address this issue, several randomized studies have compared ovarian ablation/suppression with chemotherapy alone in premenopausal women. Most of these utilized cytoxan, methotrexate, 5-fluorouracil based regimens compared with ovarian ablation/suppression.[28–32] Although none of these studies showed a statistically significant difference in outcomes, none of them was sufficiently powered to be a true equivalence trial. In addition, most of these trials included both ER-positive and ER-negative cancers, which may decrease the ability to detect an effect of ovarian ablation/suppression. Finally, most of these trials were conducted in the early 1990s when tamoxifen was not routinely given to premenopausal women, as opposed to current treatment practices.

More recently performed studies in which women were randomized either to chemotherapy alone (CMF or anthracycline-containing regimens) or ovarian ablation/suppression and tamoxifen showed similar results.[33–35] Again, most of these trials were underpowered to be considered true equivalence trials. However, the largest of these studies by the Austrian Breast Cancer Study group did demonstrate an advantage for goserelin for 3 years

Table 4.5 Effects of ovarian ablation/suppression, EBCTCG overview[7]

	Ratio of annual event rates (SE)	
	Breast cancer recurrence	Breast cancer mortality
Ovarian ablation or suppression versus nil		
Age <40 years	0.75 (0.152)	0.71 (0.13)
Age 40–49 years	0.71 (0.06)	0.71 (0.07)
Ovarian ablation/suppression + chemotherapy versus chemotherapy		
Age <40 years	0.86 (0.09)	0.96 (0.10)
Age 40–49 years	0.95 (0.07)	1.03 (0.08)

and tamoxifen for 5 years compared with CMF. It should also be noted that the women who received CMF did not receive tamoxifen, so this was not a true comparison of the effects of ovarian suppression alone.[34]

Ovarian ablation/suppression plus chemotherapy compared with chemotherapy alone

In the EBCTCG overview and three more recently conducted randomized trials, there was no additional benefit for ovarian ablation/suppression in the trials in which all women received chemotherapy.[7,31,36,37] Chemotherapy itself can induce premature menopause and therefore would interfere with the ability to detect an additional benefit of ovarian ablation/suppression. In retrospective subgroup analyses, women under the age of 40 appeared to derive greater benefit from the addition of ovarian ablation/suppression. However, these were not prospective pre-planned analyses and therefore the results would be considered as hypothesis generating, rather than truly confirmatory.

Ovarian ablation/suppression plus tamoxifen compared with tamoxifen alone

In the setting of metastatic disease, the combination of an LHRH agonist with tamoxifen was superior to tamoxifen alone in terms of response rate and progression-free and overall survival.[38] Although this issue was not directly addressed in the EBCTCG overview, combined hormonal therapy in the adjuvant setting has been addressed by two large randomized trials: an Intergroup trial that compared ovarian ablation/suppression and tamoxifen with tamoxifen alone (thus far, presented in abstract form only), and the ZIPP trial which compared goserelin (LHRH agonist) and tamoxifen with goserelin alone and tamoxifen alone.[39] Neither of these trials showed a benefit to combined hormonal therapy over either tamoxifen or ovarian suppression alone.

ADJUVANT CHEMOTHERAPY

The most comprehensive data available on the effects of adjuvant chemotherapy are those from the EBCTCG overview. As described earlier, the overview pooled centrally collected data from randomized controlled trials conducted worldwide that had started by 1995. Although covered in the overview, the role of single-agent chemotherapy as adjuvant treatment will not be discussed since this is not routinely used in current practice. In terms of polychemotherapy (including both anthracycline- and non-anthracyline-containing regimens), all women regardless of age benefited, although the absolute benefit was greater for women <50 years of age compared with women aged 50–69 years (see Figure 4.14). For women <50 years of age, polychemotherapy reduced risk of breast cancer recurrence (RR 0.63, SE 0.034, p<0.00001) and breast cancer death (RR 0.71, SE 0.040, p<0.00001), which translated to an absolute difference in 15-year breast cancer survival of 10.0%. For women aged 50–69 years, polychemotherapy also reduced the risks of breast cancer recurrence (RR 0.81, SE 0.22, p<0.0001) and breast cancer death (RR 0.88, SE 0.036, p<0.0001), translating to an absolute risk difference of 3.0% in 15-year breast cancer survival. Both node-negative and node-positive patients as a group benefited from the addition of adjuvant chemotherapy with similar proportional risk reductions. There were insufficient data to evaluate the effects of adjuvant chemotherapy in women >70 years of age. It should also be noted that most of the benefit from polychemotherapy comes from a decrease in recurrence in the first 5 years after diagnosis, although the impact on overall survival persists and grows over time. Finally, many of the women included in the trials from the EBCTCG overview were diagnosed before the widespread use of screening mammography. Although the relative benefits should be similar, the absolute benefits may be smaller with a shift towards smaller, node-negative, screen-detected tumours.

Chemohormonal therapy vs. chemotherapy alone

According to the EBCTCG overview, chemohormonal therapy (chemotherapy plus tamoxifen) was superior to tamoxifen alone in women with ER-positive tumours regardless of age (recurrence RR 0.64, SE 0.0.8 for women <50 years and RR 0.85, SE 0.04 for women 50–69 years of age, p<0.0001 for both). Therefore, tamoxifen does not seem to modify the proportional risk reduction associated with chemotherapy. Although the proportional risk reductions were the same regardless of ER status, the absolute risk difference for ER-negative disease was almost twice that of ER-positive cancers (see Figure 4.15).

However, as discussed in the guidelines above, for ER-positive cancers, chemotherapy is mainly reserved for higher risk cancer (e.g. node positive). Considerable controversy still exists as to the additional marginal benefit of chemotherapy in a postmenopausal, node-negative, ER-positive cancer. In addition, a more recently published retrospective analysis of three large CALBG randomized trials suggested that ER-positive tumours derive less benefit from the addition of anthracycline-based chemotherapy than ER-negative ones.[40]

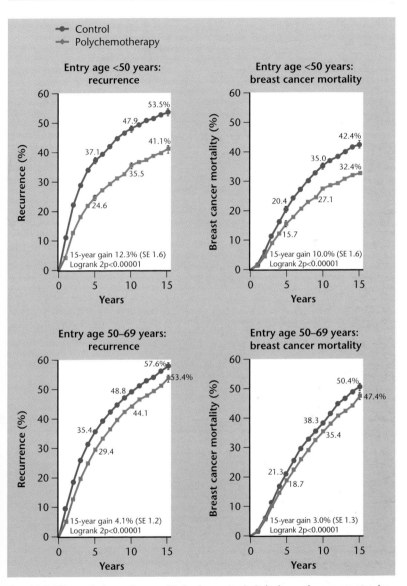

Fig. 4.14 Effects of chemotherapy (Oxford overview). Polychemotherapy vs. not, by entry age <50 or 50–69 years: 15-year probabilities of recurrence and of breast cancer mortality. Younger women, 35% node-positive; older women, 70% node-positive. Error bars are ±SE. Reproduced with permission from Early Breast Cancer Trialists' Collaborative Group (EBCTCG): Effects of chemotherapy and hormonal therapy for early breast cancer on recurrence and 15-year survival: An overview of the randomised trials. Lancet 2005; 365(9472): 1687–1717. © Elsevier Ltd.

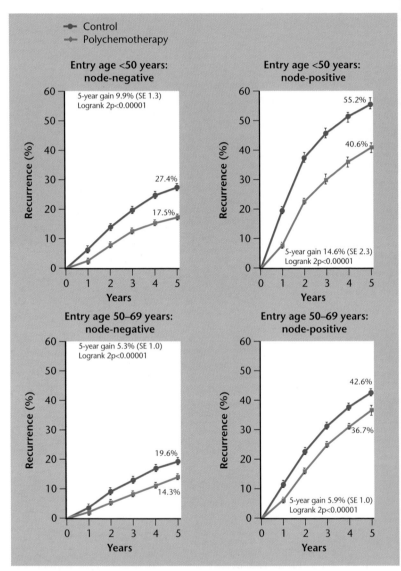

Fig. 4.15 Effects of chemotherapy by oestrogen receptor status and tamoxifen use. Polychemotherapy vs. not, by nodal status and entry age: 5-year probabilities of recurrence. Error bars are ± SE. Reproduced with permission from Early Breast Cancer Trialists' Collaborative Group (EBCTCG): Effects of chemotherapy and hormonal therapy for early breast cancer on recurrence and 15-year survival: An overview of the randomised trials. Lancet 2005; 365(9472): 1687–1717. © Elsevier Ltd.

Choice of chemotherapy

CMF vs. anthracycline-containing regimens

About one half of the trials in the overview utilized either a CMF-like regimen (cyclophosphamide (either oral or intravenous (IV)), IV methotrexate, IV 5-fluorouracil) and one-third an anthracycline-based regimen (2/3 doxorubicin and 1/3 epirubicin). Overall, the risk reduction associated with the CMF and anthracycline regimens appears similar. However, studies that directly compared CMF with anthracycline-based regimens tended to show a benefit favouring anthracylines (RR 0.89, SE 0.029, p=0.0001 for recurrence; and RR 0.84, SE 0.033, p< 0.00001 for breast cancer death favouring anthracyclines). In general, studies compared 6 months of an anthracycline (60% doxorubicin and 40% epirubicin) to 6 months of CMF. The superiority of anthracyclines was upheld across all age groups and regardless of nodal and ER status. Tables 4.6 and 4.7 give examples of the commonly used adjuvant regimens in these trials. It should be noted that the studies in the EBCTCG overview used both IV and oral CMF. IV CMF has been shown to be inferior to an anthracycline-containing regimen for node-positive cancers,[41] so the question still remains as to whether oral CMF is truly inferior to an anthraycline-containing regimen in the adjuvant setting.

Table 4.6 Commonly used anthracycline regimens (excludes taxane regimens)[166]

AC	Cyclophosphamide 600 mg/m^2 IV day 1 Doxorubicin 60 mg/m^2 IV day 1 Cycled every 21 days for 4 cycles
FAC	5-Fluorouracil 500 mg/m^2 IV days 1 and 8 Doxorubicin 50 mg/m^2 IV day 1 Cyclophosphamide 500 mg/m^2 IV day 1 Cycled every 21 days for 6 cycles
CAF	Cyclophosphamide 100 mg/m^2 PO days 1–14 Doxorubicin 30 mg/m^2 IV days 1 and 8 5-Fluorouracil 500 mg/m^2 IV days 1 and 8 Cycled every 28 days for 6 cycles
CEF	Cyclophosphamide 75 mg/m^2 PO days 1–14 Epirubicin 60 mg/m^2 IV days 1 and 8 5-Fluorouracil 500 mg/m^2 IV days 1 and 8 Cycled every 28 days for 6 cycles
EC	Epirubicin 100 mg/m^2 IV day 1 Cyclophosphamide 600 mg/m^2 IV day 1 Cycled every 21 days for 8 cycles

IV, intravenously; PO, orally

Table 4.7 CMF regimens[166]	
Oral CMF	Cyclophosphamide 100 mg/m^2 PO days 1–14 Methotrexate 40 mg/m^2 IV days 1 and 8 5-Fluorouracil 600 mg/m^2 IV days 1 and 8 Cycled every 28 days for 6 cycles
IV CMF	Cyclophosphamide 750 mg/m^2 IV day 1 Methotrexate 50 mg/m^2 IV days 1 5-Fluorouracil 600 mg/m^2 IV days 1 Cycled every 21 days for 6 cycles
IV, intravenously, PO, orally	

Retrospective analysis of several randomized trials suggested that women with Her2neu-positive cancers did not derive any benefit from the use of adjuvant CMF.[42–45] However, several other studies did not detect a difference by Her2neu status.[44] When it comes to interactions with Her2neu, the anthracyline data are much more consistent and suggest an enhanced sensitivity to anthracyclines among tumours that over-express Her2neu.[46–50] Although these interactions have not been tested prospectively, it is reasonable to consider the possible interactions when choosing an adjuvant regimen, such as favouring an anthracycline-based regimen to women with Her2neu-positive cancers. However, women with a prior history of heart disease may not be candidates for an anthracycline (please see section on side effects of chemotherapy).

Taxanes (see Table 4.8)
In the US, but less so in Europe, taxanes are also considered part of standard adjuvant chemotherapy for node-positive breast cancers. Given the recency of the taxane-based trials, they were not covered in the EBCTBG overview. Two large randomized trials (CALGB 9344 and NSABP B-28) compared doxorubicin/cyclophosphamide (AC) alone with AC and paclitaxel.[51,52] Both of these studies demonstrated a statistically significant improvement in disease-free survival although only CALGB 9344 demonstrated a statistically significant difference in overall survival (HR 0.88 favouring addition of taxane, p=0.01). As stated above, a retrospective subgroup analysis of this study suggested that ER-negative tumours were more likely to benefit from the addition of a taxane than ER positive tumours.[40]

Results from studies on docetaxel were not as clear-cut. BCIRG 001 randomized 1491 node-positive women to six cycles of FAC (see Table 4.6) or six cycles of TAC (see Table 4.8) and demonstrated a 28% reduction (p=0.001) in risk of recurrence and 30% reduction (p=0.008) in risk of

Table 4.8 Commonly used taxane regimens[166]

AC followed by T	Doxorubicin 60 mg/m² IV day 1
	Cyclophosphamide 600 mg/m² IV day 1
	Cycled every 21 days for 4 cycles followed by:
	  Paclitaxel 175 mg/m² IV by 3-hour infusion day 1
	  Cycled every 21 days for 4 cycles

Dose-dense AC-T	Doxorubicin 60 mg/m² IV day 1
	Cyclophosphamide 600 mg/m² IV day 1
	Cycled every 14 days for 4 cycles followed by:
	  Paclitaxel 175 mg/m² IV by 3 hour infusion day 1
	  Cycled every 14 days for 4 cycles
	All cycles given with growth factor support

TAC	Docetaxel 75 mg/m² IV day 1 Doxorubicin 50 mg/m² IV day 1 Cyclophosphamide 500 mg/m² IV day 1 Cycled every 21 days for 6 cycles All cycles given with growth factor support

IV, intravenously, PO, orally

death favouring TAC.[53] There was a higher risk of febrile neutropenia with TAC (25% vs. 3%, p<0.001), but no septic deaths occurred in either arm. However, another large randomized trial (NSABP B-27) that compared four cycles of AC to four cycles of AC + four cycles of docetaxel did not show any statistically significant improvement in disease-free or overall survival with the addition of docetaxel.[54,55] Again, more febrile neutropenia was seen in the docetaxel arm.

Most of the above studies limited enrollment to node-positive women, so the role of taxanes in node-negative women has not been well defined. In the US, dose-dense AC-paclitaxel has been widely adopted because of a study demonstrating superiority of the every 2 week schedule to an every 3 week schedule in terms of both disease-free and overall survival (respectively RR 0.74, p=0.01 and RR 0.69, p=0.013).[56] This must be administered with growth factor support which considerably adds to the cost of the regimen.

Trastuzumab

Approximately 20% of breast cancers over express the Her2neu protein, a tyrosine kinase like molecule that belongs to the epidermal growth factor receptor (EGFR) family.[57] Trastuzumab is a monoclonal antibody directed against the Her2neu protein. Initially studied in metastatic breast cancer, trastuzumab has now been shown to be helpful in the adjuvant treatment of breast cancer as well. At least four randomized trials have demonstrated a benefit for the addition of trastuzumab to conventional chemotherapy as adjuvant treatment in women with Her2neu-positive cancers. Tumours are considered to be Her2neu positive with a score of +3 by immunohisto-chemistry or if they show gene amplification by fluorescent *in situ* hybridization (FISH). Trastuzumab cannot be administered concurrently with doxorubicin because of an increased risk of cardiomyopathy. Cardiac function must also be monitored closely while on trastuzumab.[58,59] Several large randomized trials have reported strikingly similar results on the benefits of adjuvant trastuzumab.[60,61] All showed an approximately 50% decrease in the risk of recurrence with 1 year of adjuvant trastuzumab. The combined NSABP-Intergroup trial also found a 33% decreased risk of death (p=0.015).[61] The majority of these studies gave the trastuzumab with an anthracycline-containing regimen. The FinHer study used only 9 weeks of trastuzumab and reported similar results (RR 0.58, 95% CI 0.40–0.85, p=0.005 for recurrence or death in trastuzumab arm), consistent with the trials utilizing a full year of trastuzumab.[62]

Sequencing of chemotherapy and radiation

Adjuvant chemotherapy for breast cancer is not given concurrently with radiation because of the concerns regarding excessive toxicity with anthra-cycline-based regimens, which are widely used for breast cancer. Chemotherapy is usually given before radiation therapy because of an increased risk of distant recurrence when adjuvant chemotherapy is given afterwards. A delay of up to 6 months in order to complete adjuvant chemotherapy (for instance with the longer taxane-based regimens) has not been associated with any adverse effects on locoregional relapse, assuming that adequate margins were achieved at the time of initial surgery.[63]

Additional topics for adjuvant chemotherapy

Neoadjuvant vs. adjuvant chemotherapy

For women with locally advanced breast cancer, neoadjuvant chemotherapy, which is chemotherapy administered prior to definitive surgical resection, is often utilized. Locally advanced breast cancer includes tumours measuring >5 cm in size, involving the chest wall and/or skin, associated with bulky axillary/regional (such as supraclavic-ular) adenopathy, or inflammatory breast cancer (discussed below). There are several advantages to neoadjuvant chemotherapy including the ability to reduce tumour size, thereby improving the chances of obtaining adequate surgical margins or allowing some women the option to undergo breast-conserving surgery rather than mastectomy. Another advantage is the opportunity to evaluate *in vivo* the sensitivity of the tumour to chemotherapy agents, and modifying the regimen if the tumour does not respond. Despite these advantages, no randomized controlled trial has demonstrated a survival difference between chemotherapy administered in the neoadjvuant or adjuvant setting.[64–66]

BREAST CANCER TREATMENT IN OLDER WOMEN

Because of the higher rate of adverse side effects, poorer functional status, and competing mortality from non-breast cancer-related causes, management of breast cancer in older women remains a controversial topic. Older women should still be offered breast surgery, either lumpectomy or mastectomy and have been shown to tolerate surgery well, assuming a lack of significant comorbidities.[67] The role of axillary dissection appears to be less crucial. In both retrospective and randomized trials, there has been no significant difference in axillary failure rates and overall survival among women with ER-positive cancers and clinically node-negative axillas who took tamoxifen, but omitted axillary dissection.[68–70] In addition, several studies suggest that radiation may be omitted for elderly women who undergo breast cancer surgery and take tamoxifen. Although randomized trials have shown a higher rate of local recurrence with the omission of radiation therapy, there has been no difference in overall survival.[69,71,72] Hormone therapy with either tamoxifen or an aromatase inhibitor should be offered to women with ER-positive cancers. The additional benefit of chemotherapy has not been well defined in this group. The EBCTBG and most randomized trials have contained too few women over the age of 70 to make any definitive recommendations. For tumours that are ER negative or node positive and ER positive, it is reasonable to consider chemotherapy in a woman without significant comorbidity with a long enough life expectancy to enjoy the potential benefits and lower likelihood of adverse effects from chemotherapy. Adjuvant! Online can also be helpful at estimating risks and benefits since the program takes into account a person's age and comorbidity from competing causes when estimating disease-free and overall survival.

LONG-TERM SIDE EFFECTS OF CHEMOTHERAPY

When deciding upon the risks and benefits of adjuvant chemotherapy, one needs to consider the possibility of long-term side effects. Although less common than short-term side effects such as alopecia, gastrointestinal upset and immunosuppression, these long-term side effects may significantly impact a person who is otherwise cured of breast cancer.

PREMATURE MENOPAUSE

Although temporary chemotherapy-induced amenorrhoea is common among all women, some women who were premenopausal prior to chemotherapy will undergo permanent premature ovarian failure as a direct result of the treatment. This percentage depends upon both the type of chemotherapy and the age of the patient at treatment. CMF or CEF-like regimens are more commonly associated with premature menopause than AC-like regimens. Premature menopause also becomes more common in older compared with younger women.[73-75]

CARDIAC TOXICITY

The two drugs used in adjuvant treatment of breast cancer most commonly associated with cardiac toxicity are doxorubicin and trastuzumab. The risk of cardiomyopathy with doxorubicin is related to both age and cumulative dose. For example, in a pooled analysis of three randomized controlled trials the cumulative percentage of congestive heart failure at 300 mg/m^2, 400 mg/m^2, 500 mg/m^2 and 600 mg/m^2 was 1.7%, 4.7%, 15.7% and 32.4% respectively among all patients. In addition, patients older than 65 years were more than twice as likely to experience congestive heart failure compared with younger patients. The dose of doxorubicin used in most standard regimens (240–300 mg/m^2) is associated with a 1–2% risk of symptomatic congestive heart failure.[76] In the adjuvant trastuzumab trials, the addition of trastuzumab increased the risk of symptomatic congestive heart failure compared with chemotherapy alone (2–4% for trastuzumab + chemotherapy compared with 0–1% for chemotherapy alone).[60-62]

LEUKAEMIA AND MYELODYSPLASTIC SYNDROME

Both cyclophosphamide- and doxorubicin-containing regimens have been associated with a low risk (<1%) of secondary myeloid leukaemias/myelodysplastic syndrome when given at standard adjuvant doses. However, these treatment-related leukaemias may be more refractory to treatment and associated with a poorer prognosis.[77]

METASTATIC DISEASE

Although the majority of women present with disease localized to the breast and axillary lymph nodes, some women will go on to develop systemic metastases. The risk of systemic metastases is highest within the first 10 years of diagnosis, but it is not uncommon for women to relapse more than 10 years after diagnosis.[78] Metastatic breast cancer can have a variable natural history with a median survival of approximately 2 years, but with a wide range and a few percent considered 'long-term' survivors (greater than 10 years). However, the majority of women with metastatic disease will die of metastatic disease. Therefore, the goals of treatment differ from those of adjuvant therapy in which women may potentially be cured of breast cancer.

MONITORING OF RESPONSE AND GOALS OF TREATMENT

There are no prospective randomized trials proving the benefit of chemotherapy over observation alone, so the goals of therapy are palliative. However, several criteria can be used to monitor clinical utility and response to treatment. Response rate (usually documented as changes in radiographic measurements of metastases) is frequently used for clinical trials, although this may underestimate the benefits of treatment. A patient may notice improvement in quality of life without large radiographic differences. In addition, radiographically stable disease can also be associated with similar overall survival to those who achieve a complete or partial radiographic response.[79] Physical exam can also be used to quantitate response for those women with easily measurable disease such as skin nodules.

Since palliation is the main goal of treatment, assessment of symptoms due to cancer, such as pain and fatigue, are helpful. In clinical trials, different scales to measure quality of life are also utilized.

Tumour markers such as CA 27-29 (or CA 15-3) and carcinoembryonic antigen (CEA) can sometimes be helpful in monitoring response, giving better correlation with disease response with CA 27-29.[80,81] However, tumour markers alone should not be the sole determinant of treatment response. Tumour markers can transiently increase ('flare' response) soon after initiating treatment.[82] Levels may also be elevated due to non-neoplastic causes, such as hepatic disease or megaloblastic anaemia.[83,84] In addition, some women with metastatic breast may have normal tumour markers.

Although radiation and surgery can also serve important palliative roles as well, the following discussion will centre on systemic treatment options since the focus of this handbook is on medical management of breast cancer.

HORMONAL THERAPY FOR METASTATIC BREAST CANCER

In general, women with hormone-sensitive breast cancer, lower disease burden and minimum symptoms due to breast cancer should be treated with hormonal therapy first. Other factors predictive of a response to hormonal therapy include a longer disease-free interval, bone-only disease, lack of bulky visceral involvement, and prior response to hormonal therapy. Although some data suggest the Her2neu status may modify response to hormonal therapy, it is still reasonable to consider a trial of hormonal therapy alone first in someone with hormone-sensitive Her2neu-positive cancer. Hormonal therapy and chemotherapy are usually tried sequentially rather than concurrently, since there is no large survival benefit to combination therapy.[85]

Postmenopausal women

High-dose oestrogen and progesterones were used for the treatment of metastatic breast cancer until the introduction in the 1970s of tamoxifen, which is now being supplanted by AI. Either tamoxifen or an AI would be considered reasonable first-line hormonal treatment for metastatic breast cancer in a woman who has not previously received the drug. Compared with tamoxifen, AI are associated with a slight improvement in response rate and time to progression.[86,87] For progression after an AI, tamoxifen can be considered, and the converse for women who began on an AI. In general, re-treatment with an agent already given in the adjuvant setting is not done. For women who progress after both an AI and tamoxifen and still remain candidates for hormonal therapy, treatment with an anti-oestrogen such as fulvestrant can be considered. High-dose oestrogen and progesterone are occasionally used, but women must be aware of the risks of thromboembolic events and weight gain. Discussions of specific agents follow below.

Premenopausal women

For premenopausal women, first-line hormonal therapy consists of tamoxifen and ovarian suppression/ablation, depending upon whether either treatment has already been utilized. Similar to the adjuvant setting, ovarian suppression can be achieved pharmacologically using an LHRH agonist or ovarian ablation through surgery or radiation. For women not previously on tamoxifen, tamoxifen combined with ovarian suppression can be associated with higher response rates and improvement in disease-free and overall survival compared with tamoxifen alone.[38] AI cannot be used alone in premenopausal women because the decrease in oestrogen level can increase gonatropin secretion from the pituitary/hypothalamus, leading to ovarian stimulation. However, the combination of an LHRH agonist and AI can be associated with reasonable clinical response.[88]

Tamoxifen and other SERMs

Tamoxifen at 20 mg daily can be used in both premenopausal and post-menopausal women. Please see the adjuvant section for a discussion of adverse events associated with tamoxifen. In a minority of patients who begin tamoxifen for metastatic cancer, a 'flare' response can be observed with an increase in bone pain and/or skin nodules within the first month of beginning treatment due to tamoxifen's partial agonist activity. Accompanying radiographic changes suggesting disease progression can also be observed. Symptoms should resolve within 1 month.[89] A withdrawal response upon discontinuation of tamoxifen can also occasionally be observed.[90]

In addition to tamoxifen, toremifene has also been approved in the US for the treatment of metastatic breast cancer. Clinical activity and response rates are similar to tamoxifen.[91] However, it has little activity in women with tamoxifen-resistant disease.[92]

Aromatase inhibitors

Currently, three aromatase inhibitors (anastrozole, letrozole, and exemestane) are used to treat breast cancer in the adjuvant and metastatic settings. Anastrozole and letrozole are non-steroidal reversible AI whereas exemestane is a steroidal irreversible AI. All three strongly suppress circulating oestradiol and oestrone and can be utilized in the first-line setting or in tamoxifen-resistant disease.[93–95] Clinically, there does not appear to be any significant difference among the three. Letrozole was directly compared with anastrazole as second-line hormonal therapy with a slight increase in response rate, but no difference in overall survival, time to progression or clinical benefit.[96] Exemestane also shows some activity in disease refractory to a non-steroidal AI[97,98] and the converse is true as well.[98]

Other hormonal therapies

Fulvestrant is a pure oestrogen antagonist administered monthly by intramuscular injection, with demonstrated activity in tamoxifen-resistant[99,100] and AI-resistant advanced breast cancer.[101] Progestins, such as megestrol acetate 40 mg qid, are also active, but have more side effects than either tamoxifen or the AI.

CHEMOTHERAPY FOR METASTATIC BREAST CANCER

Initial response rates for first-line chemotherapy regimens in metastatic breast cancer are approximately 50–75%. For women with Her2neu-positive cancers, trastuzumab can be used in place of or in addition to chemotherapy. Please see the section below on trastuzumab for more details.

Choice of chemotherapy

Many different chemotherapies have been associated with reasonable response rates as single agents, including paclitaxel, docetaxel, vinorelbine, gemcitabine, capecitabine, doxorubicin, liposomal doxorubicin, albumin-bound paclitaxel and etoposide. In general, the taxanes and anthracyclines have been utilized most often in the first- or second-line setting with no clear superiority for one over the other.[102,103] The same drugs given in the adjuvant setting are not generally recommended as first-line therapy for women with metastatic disease with a disease-free period of less than 12 months after treatment. In addition, the cumulative anthracycline exposure should be calculated in a woman who received an anthracycline in the adjuvant setting. As for the choice of taxanes, docetaxel may be a slightly more active drug than paclitaxel in the metastatic setting but paclitaxel is better tolerated.[104] Therefore, either would be considered a reasonable option.

Singlet vs. doublet chemotherapy

Multiple doublet regimens (e.g. doxorubicin + pacliaxel, carboplatin + docetaxel) have been compared with treatment with a single agent. In general, the doublet regimens are associated with a higher response rate and longer times to progression, but this is offset by a higher rate of adverse side effects and modest, if any, difference in overall survival.[85,105] However, many of these studies compared the doublet regimen with a sole single agent, rather than the doublet with sequential therapy with both of the agents given alone. Two trials which directly compared concurrent treatment with sequential single agent treatment showed no significant difference in overall survival.[106,107] Thus, in general, sequential single-agent therapy would be reasonable for the treatment of metastatic breast cancer, with doublet chemotherapy reserved for those with rapidly progressive symptomatic visceral disease who may benefit from the slightly higher response rate with the doublet regimens.

High-dose chemotherapy

High-dose chemotherapy with stem cell support has been evaluated for the treatment of metastatic breast cancer and there has been no consistent evidence for any significant difference in disease-free or overall survival.[108] Therefore, high-dose chemotherapy should only be considered within the context of a clinical trial.

BIOLOGICAL THERAPIES

Biological therapies is a somewhat loose term, but generally refers to treatment with mechanisms of action that differ from standard hormonal or chemotherapy.

Trastuzumab

The most extensively studied of the biological agents for breast cancer is trastuzumab. As described in the adjuvant treatment section, trastuzumab is a monoclonal antibody directed against the Her2neu protein, a tyrosine kinase-like molecule belonging to the EGFR family. Her2neu is over-expressed in about 20% of breast cancers.[57] Treatment with trastuzumab should be reserved for those tumours with high levels of expression (+3) by immunohistochemistry or demonstrating gene amplification by FISH. As both a single agent and in combination with chemotherapy, trastuzumab has been associated with excellent response rates. As monotherapy, it can be administered intravenously either weekly (2 mg/kg) or every 3 weeks (6 mg/kg), following the administration of a loading dose (4 mg/kg for weekly therapy and 8 mg/kg for every 3-week therapy). It should be noted that trastuzumab does not cross the blood-brain barrier, so the central nervous system is a frequent site of progressive disease in someone with Her2neu-positive cancer on trastuzumab.[109,110]

Given preclinical data suggesting synergy between trastuzumab and chemotherapy, trastuzumab is widely given concurrently with chemotherapy. Outside clinical trials, trastuzumab is not given concurrently with an anthracycline because of the increased risk of heart failure.[58] Trastuzumab has been given in combination with several other chemotherapy agents, including paclitaxel,[58] docetaxel,[111–113] carboplatin[114,115] and vinorelbine.[116,117] The duration of trastuzumab therapy after progression after treatment with a trastuzumab-containing regimen is still not known.

Lapatinib

Another way to block Her2neu would be via tyrosine kinase inhibition. Lapatinib is an oral dual inhibitor of both EGFR and Her2neu tyrosine kinases. A randomized controlled trial demonstrated a statistically significant improvement in time to progression for lapatinib and capecitabine, compared with capecitabine alone.[117a] Activity was also seen in trastuzumab-resistant breast cancer.[118]

Bevacizumab

Another promising biological agent with activity in breast cancer is bevacizumab, a monoclonal antibody directed against vascular endothelial growth factor. Although it has only modest activity as a single agent, a preliminary report in abstract form suggested that the response rate and progression-free survival improved when combined with paclitaxel. However, there was a higher incidence of hypertension, proteinuria and bleeding complications in the bevacizumab arm. Bevacizumab is also contraindicated in patients with a history of brain metastases, due to a higher risk of haemorrhagic complications.

Bisphosphonates

In randomized controlled trials, monthly intravenous bisphosphonates have been shown to decrease the risk of skeletal complications compared with placebo in women with breast cancer metastatic to bone.[119] The two most widely used in metastatic breast cancer are pamidronate and zoledronate. These are considerably more potent than the oral biphosphonates. Serum creatinine and calcium should be monitored on bisphophonates.

ADDITIONAL TOPICS

BREAST CANCER DURING PREGNANCY

Breast cancer during pregnancy is relatively uncommon, affecting between 1 in 3,000 and 1 in 10,000 pregnancies in the US, representing only a few percent of the breast cancers diagnosed in women under the age of 50 years.[120–122] Due to pregnancy's effects on the breast, it can be difficult to distinguish between benign and malignant findings in the breast solely using physical exam. Diagnostic delays of several months are quite common in pregnancy-associated breast cancer.[122] Ultrasound is usually the first diagnostic test, since this avoids fetal radiation exposure. Mammography can also be performed with abdominal shielding with only minimal fetal radiation exposure. Since gadolinium should be avoided during pregnancy, diagnostic breast magnetic resonance imaging (MRI) is not usually performed.[123] Fine-needle aspiration, core needle biopsies and surgical biopsies can all be performed safely during pregnancy with local anaesthesia. Staging scans such as ultrasounds and plain radiographs with proper shielding, can be performed during pregnancy. Computed tomography (CT) scans should be avoided because of the larger dose of radiation. Partly due to delays in diagnosis, breast cancers diagnosed during pregnancy tend towards larger size and more advanced stage.[124–126]

Breast and axillary surgery can be performed safely during pregnancy, with the recognition that adjuvant radiation therapy is contraindicated during pregnancy. In general, most of the chemotherapy agents used in breast cancer can be safely administered in either the second or third trimester, with the exception of methotrexate which is an abortifacent.[127] The most commonly used agents are cyclophosphamide and doxorubicin +/– 5-fluouracil, which has been evaluated prospectively in pregnant women.[128] Few data exist on the safety of trastuzumab during pregnancy. Tamoxifen should be avoided because of associations with birth defects and fetal death.[129]

Most studies have found that pregnancy was not an independent adverse prognostic factor, after controlling for stage.[124,125,130,131] Although there may be an increased risk of premature birth, there does not appear to be any long-term adverse effect of chemotherapy administration on the child.[128,132]

IN SITU DISEASE

The prognosis for patients with *in situ* lesions is very good. Nonetheless, invasive lesions will develop in a certain fraction of patients with *in situ* carcinomas. Surgery, as either a mastectomy or breast-conserving surgery + adjuvant radiotherapy, has been the treatment of choice for ductal carcinoma *in situ* (DCIS) lesions.[133,134] In addition to local therapies, tamoxifen may decrease the risk of recurrence by approximately 50%,[135] although this effect of tamoxifen was not seen in a large European trial.[136] When DCIS does recur, about half of the recurrences are invasive and half non-invasive.[133] DCIS represents a rather heterogeneous group. One common general principle is attaining adequate surgical margins (at least 1 cm). In general, radiation therapy would be added for women who had breast-conserving surgery although wide excision alone can be considered for smaller, lower-grade lesions with wide surgical margins. Tamoxifen can be considered, although the data are inconsistent and no survival difference has been shown.

Management options for lobular carcinoma *in situ* (LCIS) include careful observation, bilateral prophylactic simple mastectomy or the use of tamoxifen.

INFLAMMATORY BREAST CANCER

Inflammatory breast cancer (IBC) is a specific subset of locally advanced breast cancer. IBC is relatively rare, comprises only 1–2% of all breast cancers, and is more common in black women than white women.[137] The classic histological finding is invasion of the dermal lymphatics by tumour cells. However, this is not absolutely necessary and a diagnosis can also be made on clinical grounds. The typical presentation would be a rapidly enlarging mass associated with erythema of the skin and brawny induration, described as 'peau d'orange' (skin of an orange). Initially, IBC can be mistaken for a mastitis or cellulitis. Mammography may not necessarily show a well-defined mass. It is crucial to stage these women at diagnosis since approximately one-third may present with distant metastases.[138] Treatment for locally advanced breast cancer involves neoadjuvant chemotherapy (as described previously), surgery and radiation therapy.

METASTATIC BREAST CANCER IN AN AXILLARY LYMPH NODE

Women who present with adenocarcinoma in an axillary lymph node without clinical evidence of a primary breast cancer should undergo thorough evaluation for an occult breast primary, including diagnostic mammography and MRI, if a mammogram is normal. If appropriate, these women can also be considered for breast-conserving surgery.

If a primary breast cancer cannot be identified, an axillary dissection should still be performed for purposes of local control. The role of breast surgery is somewhat controversial, although the risk of breast recurrence is higher in the absence of mastectomy. Irradiation of the breast can be considered in lieu of mastectomy.[139–141] Adjuvant systemic treatment follows guidelines for node-positive breast cancer.

MALE BREAST CANCER

Male breast cancer is much less common than female breast cancer. Median age at diagnosis is approximately 65 years.[142,143] Male breast cancer can also be associated with mutations in *BRCA1* or *BRCA2*, although the association is stronger for *BRCA2*.[144,145] The majority of male invasive breast cancers are ductal and hormone sensitive.[146,147] Staging and principles of treatment are similar to those in women with breast cancer, except that tamoxifen is preferred over AI which seem to have limited utility in male breast cancer.[147,148]

CENTRAL NERVOUS SYSTEM INVOLVEMENT IN METASTATIC BREAST CANCER

Brain metastases

Although less common as a first site of metastatic involvement, clinically apparent brain metastases affect approximately 10% of women with metastatic breast cancer and are more common among women with Her2neu positive cancers.[149–151] Signs and symptoms are variable and can include headaches, focal neurological deficits, seizures or nausea and vomiting. Corticosteroids can provide symptomatic relief by decreasing peri-tumoral oedema. Anticonvulsants are given to those with seizures, but do not necessarily need to be given to all women with brain metastases prophylactically.[152,153] Options for definitive treatment of brain metastases include whole-brain radiation therapy, stereotactic radiosurgery, and neurosurgery. The choice among these options should be individualized according to the patient's overall prognosis, performance status, age and extent of visceral involvement.

Epidural metastases

Untreated epidural metastases can leave significant functional deficits, so a high suspicion for epidural involvement in a woman with metastatic breast cancer must always be maintained. Back pain is the most common presenting symptom. Eventually, progressive motor and sensory deficits will develop, then incontinence. For diagnosis, MRI is preferred over CT because of superior imaging of the epidural space. Corticosteroids can help with pain and neurological symptoms. Urgent institution of radiation is crucial to preserving function. Outcome after treatment is directly related to the patient's functional status at the time of treatment. Patients who are ambulatory before treatment generally remain so. However, only a minority of patients who are paraplegic can walk after radiation and/or surgery, emphasizing the importance of rapid diagnosis and treatment.[154–157] In one randomized controlled trial enrolling patients with a variety of cancers, immediate surgery was superior to radiation in preserving the ability to walk.[158] However, it is not clear if these results would apply to institutions where immediate neurosurgery may not be available and to breast cancer which is among the more radiosensitive tumours.

Leptomeningeal metastases

Leptomeningeal involvement, also called carcinomatous meninigitis, occurs when breast cancer spreads to the subarachnoid space and/or cerebrospinal fluid (CSF). Patients will generally present with multifocal neurological abnormalities, such as spinal symptoms (e.g. leg weakness), cranial nerve abnormalities, or symptoms suggestive of CSF obstruction (e.g. headaches, nausea and vomiting). Diagnosis can be made with MRI with gadolinium showing leptomeningeal or cranial nerve enhancement. However, MRI is negative in about 10% of people with solid tumours and leptomeningeal involvement. In those situations, a lumbar puncture will need to be performed to obtain CSF cytology.[159,160] CSF protein is usually elevated. The sensitivity of a single lumbar puncture for detecting leptomeningeal involvement is about 50%, but increases to more than 90% after three taps.[161] Prognosis is typically poor with median survival of 4–6 months so treatment should be directed towards symptomatic disease. The entire neuraxis should be imaged and symptomatic or bulky areas should be irradiated. Systemic chemotherapy is minimally helpful for treatment because of the blood-brain barrier, so intrathecal chemotherapy can be considered. Intrathecal chemotherapy with activity in breast cancer includes methotrexate, thiotepa and cytarabine.[162–164] However, it is not clear that intrathecal therapy provides any survival benefit over supportive care alone.

REFERENCES

1. Ravdin PM, Siminoff LA, et al: Computer program to assist in making decisions about adjuvant therapy for women with early breast cancer. J Clin Oncol 2001; 19(4): 980–991.
2. Olivotto IA, Bajdik CD, et al: Population-based validation of the prognostic model ADJUVANT! for early breast cancer. J Clin Oncol 2005; 23(12): 2716–2725.
3. Paik S, Shak S, et al: A multigene assay to predict recurrence of tamoxifen-treated, node-negative breast cancer. N Engl J Med 2004; 351(27): 2817–2826.
4. Esteva FJ, Sahin AA, et al: Prognostic role of a multigene reverse transcriptase-PCR assay in patients with node-negative breast cancer not receiving adjuvant systemic therapy. Clin Cancer Res 2005; 11(9): 3315–3319.
5. Paik S, Tang G, et al: Gene expression and benefit of chemotherapy in women with node-negative, estrogen receptor-positive breast cancer. J Clin Oncol 2006; 24(23): 3726–3734.
6. Paik S. Molecular profiling of breast cancer. Curr Opin Obstet Gynecol 2006; 18(1): 59–63.
7. Early Breast Cancer Trialists' Collaborative Group (EBCTCG): Effects of chemotherapy and hormonal therapy for early breast cancer on recurrence and 15-year survival: an overview of the randomised trials. Lancet 2005; 365(9472): 1687–1717.
8. Fisher B, Dignam J, Bryant J, Wolmark N: Five versus more than five years of tamoxifen for lymph node-negative breast cancer: updated findings from the National Surgical Adjuvant Breast and Bowel Project B-14 randomized trial. J Natl Cancer Inst 2001; 93(9): 684–690.

9. Stewart HJ, Prescott RJ, et al: Scottish adjuvant tamoxifen trial: A randomized study updated to 15 years. J Natl Cancer Inst 2001; 93(6): 456–462.

10. Tormey DC, Gray R, et al: Postchemotherapy adjuvant tamoxifen therapy beyond five years in patients with lymph node-positive breast cancer. Eastern Cooperative Oncology Group. J Natl Cancer Inst 1996; 88(24): 1828–1833.

11. Albain KS, Green SJ, et al: Adjuvant chemohormonal therapy for primary breast cancer should be sequential instead of concurrent: Initial results from intergroup trial 0100 (SWOG-8814). Proc ASCO 2002; 21: 37a.

12. Pico C, Martin M, et al: Epirubicin-cyclophosphamide adjuvant chemotherapy plus tamoxifen administered concurrently versus sequentially: randomized phase III trial in postmenopausal node-positive breast cancer patients. A GEICAM 9401 study. Ann Oncol 2004; 15(1): 79–87.

13. Wazer DE, Tercilla OF, et al: Modulation in the radiosensitivity of MCF-7 human breast carcinoma cells by 17B-estradiol and tamoxifen. Br J Radiol 1989; 62(744): 1079–1083.

14. Paulsen GH, Strickert T, et al: Changes in radiation sensitivity and steroid receptor content induced by hormonal agents and ionizing radiation in breast cancer cells in vitro. Acta Oncol 1996; 35(8): 1011–1019.

15. Ahn PH, Vu HT, et al: Sequence of radiotherapy with tamoxifen in conservatively managed breast cancer does not affect local relapse rates. J Clin Oncol 2005; 23(1): 17–23.

16. Harris EE, Christensen VJ, et al: Impact of concurrent versus sequential tamoxifen with radiation therapy in early-stage breast cancer patients undergoing breast conservation treatment. J Clin Oncol 2005; 23(1): 11–16.

17. Pierce LJ, Hutchins LF, et al: Sequencing of tamoxifen and radiotherapy after breast-conserving surgery in early-stage breast cancer. J Clin Oncol 2005; 23(1): 24–29.

18. Fisher B, Costantino JP, et al: Tamoxifen for the prevention of breast cancer: Current status of the National Surgical Adjuvant Breast and Bowel Project P-1 study. J Natl Cancer Inst 2005; 97(22): 1652–1662.

19. Cuzick J, Powles T, et al: Overview of the main outcomes in breast-cancer prevention trials. Lancet 2003; 361(9354): 296–300.

20. Baum M, Budzar AU, et al: Anastrozole alone or in combination with tamoxifen versus tamoxifen alone for adjuvant treatment of postmenopausal women with early breast cancer: First results of the ATAC randomised trial. Lancet 2002; 359(9324): 2131–2139.

21. Howell A, Cuzick J, et al: Results of the ATAC (Arimidex, Tamoxifen, Alone or in Combination) trial after completion of 5 years' adjuvant treatment for breast cancer. Lancet 2005; 365(9453): 60–62.

22. Thurlimann B, Keshaviah A, et al: A comparison of letrozole and tamoxifen in postmenopausal women with early breast cancer. N Engl J Med 2005; 353(26): 2747–2757.

23. Goss PE, Ingle JN, et al: A randomized trial of letrozole in postmenopausal women after five years of tamoxifen therapy for early-stage breast cancer. N Engl J Med 2003; 349(19): 1793–1802.

24. Goss PE, Ingle JN, et al: Randomized trial of letrozole following tamoxifen as extended adjuvant therapy in receptor-positive breast cancer: Updated findings from NCIC CTG MA.17. J Natl Cancer Inst 2005; 97(17): 1262–1271.

25. Coombes RC, Hall E, et al: A randomized trial of exemestane after two to three years of tamoxifen therapy in postmenopausal women with primary breast cancer. N Engl J Med 2004; 350(11): 1081–1092.

26. Jakesz R, Jonat W, et al: Switching of postmenopausal women with endocrine-responsive early breast cancer to anastrozole after 2 years' adjuvant tamoxifen: Combined results of ABCSG trial 8 and ARNO 95 trial. Lancet 2005; 366(9484): 455–462.

27. Boccardo F, Rubagotti A, et al: Switching to anastrozole versus continued tamoxifen treatment of early breast cancer. Updated results of the Italian tamoxifen anastrozole (ITA) trial. Ann Oncol 2006; 17 Suppl 7: vii10–vii14.

28. Scottish Cancer Trials Breast Group and ICRF Breast Unit, Guy's Hospital, London: Adjuvant ovarian ablation versus CMF chemotherapy in premenopausal women with pathological stage II breast carcinoma: The Scottish trial. Lancet 1993; 341(8856): 1293–1298.

29. Jonat W, Kaufmann M, et al: Goserelin versus cyclophosphamide, methotrexate, and fluorouracil as adjuvant therapy in premenopausal patients with node-positive breast cancer: The Zoladex Early Breast Cancer Research Association Study. J Clin Oncol 2002; 20(24): 4628–4635.

30. Schmid P, Untch M, et al: Cyclophosphamide, methotrexate and fluorouracil (CMF) versus hormonal ablation with leuprorelin acetate as adjuvant treatment of node-positive, premenopausal breast cancer patients: Preliminary results of the TABLE-study (Takeda Adjuvant Breast cancer study with Leuprorelin Acetate). Anticancer Res 2002; 22(4): 2325–2332.

31. Castiglione-Gertsch M, O'Neill A, et al: Adjuvant chemotherapy followed by goserelin versus either modality alone for premenopausal lymph node-negative breast cancer: A randomized trial. J Natl Cancer Inst 2003; 95(24): 1833–1846.

32. Kaufmann M, Jonat W, et al: Survival analyses from the ZEBRA study. goserelin (Zoladex) versus CMF in premenopausal women with node-positive breast cancer. Eur J Cancer 2003; 39(12): 1711–1717.

33. Boccardo F, Rubagotti A, et al: Cyclophosphamide, methotrexate, and fluorouracil versus tamoxifen plus ovarian suppression as adjuvant treatment of estrogen receptor-positive pre-/perimenopausal breast cancer patients: Results of the Italian Breast Cancer Adjuvant Study Group 02 randomized trial. boccardo@hp380.ist.unige.it. J Clin Oncol 2000; 18(14): 2718–2727.

34. Jakesz R, Hausmaninger H, et al: Randomized adjuvant trial of tamoxifen and goserelin versus cyclophosphamide, methotrexate, and fluorouracil: Evidence for the superiority of treatment with endocrine blockade in premenopausal patients with hormone-responsive breast cancer—Austrian Breast and Colorectal Cancer Study Group Trial 5. J Clin Oncol 2002; 20(24): 4621–4627.

35. Roche H, Kerbrat P, et al: Complete hormonal blockade versus epirubicin-based chemotherapy in premenopausal, one to three node-positive, and hormone-receptor positive, early breast cancer patients: 7-year follow-up results of French Adjuvant Study Group 06 randomised trial. Ann Oncol 2006; 17(8): 1221–1227.

36. Arriagada R, Le MG, et al: Randomized trial of adjuvant ovarian suppression in 926 premenopausal patients with early breast cancer treated with adjuvant chemotherapy. Ann Oncol 2005; 16(3): 389–396.

37. Davidson NE, O'Neill AM, et al: Chemoendocrine therapy for premenopausal women with axillary lymph node-positive, steroid hormone receptor-positive breast cancer: Results from INT 0101 (E5188). J Clin Oncol 2005; 23(25): 5973–5982.

38. Klijn JG, Blamey RW, et al: Combined tamoxifen and luteinizing hormone-releasing hormone (LHRH) agonist versus LHRH agonist alone in premenopausal advanced breast cancer: A meta-analysis of four randomized trials. J Clin Oncol 2001; 19(2): 343–353.

39. Baum M, Hackshaw A, et al: Adjuvant goserelin in pre-menopausal patients with early breast cancer: Results from the ZIPP study. Eur J Cancer 2006; 42(7): 895–904.

40. Berry DA, Cirrincione C, et al: Estrogen-receptor status and outcomes of modern chemotherapy for patients with node-positive breast cancer. JAMA 2006; 295(14): 1658–1667.

41. Coombes RC, Bliss JM, et al: Adjuvant cyclophosphamide, methotrexate, and fluorouracil versus fluorouracil, epirubicin, and cyclophosphamide chemotherapy in premenopausal women with axillary node-positive operable breast cancer: Results of a randomized trial. The International Collaborative Cancer Group. J Clin Oncol 1996; 14(1): 35–45.

42. Allred DC, Clark GM, et al: HER-2/neu in node-negative breast cancer: Prognostic significance of overexpression influenced by the presence of in situ carcinoma. J Clin Oncol 1992; 10(4): 599–605.

43. Gusterson BA, Gelber RD, et al: Prognostic importance of c-erbB-2 expression in breast cancer. International (Ludwig) Breast Cancer Study Group. J Clin Oncol 1992; 10(7): 1049–1056.

44. Miles DW, Harris WH, et al: Effect of c-erbB(2) and estrogen receptor status on survival of women with primary breast cancer treated with adjuvant cyclophosphamide/methotrexate/fluorouracil. Int J Cancer 1999; 84(4): 354–359.

45. Moliterni A, Menard S, et al: HER2 overexpression and doxorubicin in adjuvant chemotherapy for resectable breast cancer. J Clin Oncol 2003; 21(3): 458–462.

46. Paik S, Bryant J, et al: erbB-2 and response to doxorubicin in patients with axillary lymph node-positive, hormone receptor-negative breast cancer. J Natl Cancer Inst 1998; 90(18): 1361–1370.

47. Thor AD, Berry DA, et al: erbB-2, p53, and efficacy of adjuvant therapy in lymph node-positive breast cancer. J Natl Cancer Inst 1998; 90(18): 1346–1360.

48. Paik S, Bryant J, et al: HER2 and choice of adjuvant chemotherapy for invasive breast cancer: National Surgical Adjuvant Breast and Bowel Project Protocol B-15. J Natl Cancer Inst 2000; 92(24): 1991–1998.

49. Del Mastro L, Bruzzi P, et al: HER2 expression and efficacy of dose-dense anthracycline-containing adjuvant chemotherapy in breast cancer patients. Br J Cancer 2005; 93(1): 7–14.

50. Pritchard KI, Shepherd LE, et al: HER2 and responsiveness of breast cancer to adjuvant chemotherapy. N Engl J Med 2006; 354(20): 2103–2111.

51. Henderson IC, Berry DA, et al: Improved outcomes from adding sequential paclitaxel but not from escalating doxorubicin dose in an adjuvant chemotherapy regimen for patients with node-positive primary breast cancer. J Clin Oncol 2003; 21(6): 976–983.

52. Mamounas EP, Bryant J, et al: Paclitaxel after doxorubicin plus cyclophosphamide as adjuvant chemotherapy for node-positive breast cancer: results from NSABP B-28. J Clin Oncol 2005; 23(16): 3686–3696.

53. Martin M, Pienkowski T, et al: Adjuvant docetaxel for node-positive breast cancer. N Engl J Med 2005; 352(22): 2302–2313.

54. Bear HD, Anderson S, et al: The effect on tumor response of adding sequential preoperative docetaxel to preoperative doxorubicin and cyclophosphamide: Preliminary results from National Surgical Adjuvant Breast and Bowel Project Protocol B-27. J Clin Oncol 2003; 21(22): 4165–4174.

55. Bear HD, Anderson S, et al: Sequential preoperative or postoperative docetaxel added to preoperative doxorubicin plus cyclophosphamide for operable breast cancer: National Surgical Adjuvant Breast and Bowel Project Protocol B-27. J Clin Oncol 2006; 24(13): 2019–2027.
56. Citron ML, Berry DA, et al: Randomized trial of dose-dense versus conventionally scheduled and sequential versus concurrent combination chemotherapy as postoperative adjuvant treatment of node-positive primary breast cancer: First report of Intergroup Trial C9741/Cancer and Leukemia Group B Trial 9741. J Clin Oncol 2003; 21(8): 1431–1439.
57. Klapper LN, Glathe S, et al: The ErbB-2/HER2 oncoprotein of human carcinomas may function solely as a shared coreceptor for multiple stroma-derived growth factors. Proc Natl Acad Sci U S A 1999; 96(9): 4995–5000.
58. Slamon DJ, Leyland-Jones B, et al: Use of chemotherapy plus a monoclonal antibody against HER2 for metastatic breast cancer that overexpresses HER2. N Engl J Med 2001; 344(11): 783–792.
59. Seidman A, Hudis C, et al: Cardiac dysfunction in the trastuzumab clinical trials experience. J Clin Oncol 2002; 20(5): 1215–1221.
60. Piccart-Gebhart MJ, Procter M, et al: Trastuzumab after adjuvant chemotherapy in HER2-positive breast cancer. N Engl J Med 2005; 353(16): 1659–1672.
61. Romond EH, Perez EA, et al: Trastuzumab plus adjuvant chemotherapy for operable HER2-positive breast cancer. N Engl J Med 2005; 353(16): 1673–1684.
62. Joensuu H, Kellokumpu-Lehtinen PL, et al: Adjuvant docetaxel or vinorelbine with or without trastuzumab for breast cancer. N Engl J Med 2006; 354(8): 809–820.
63. Sartor CI, Peterson BL, et al: Effect of addition of adjuvant paclitaxel on radiotherapy delivery and locoregional control of node-positive breast cancer: cancer and leukemia group B 9344. J Clin Oncol 2005; 23(1): 30–40.
64. Fisher B, Bryant J, et al: Effect of preoperative chemotherapy on the outcome of women with operable breast cancer. J Clin Oncol 1998; 16(8): 2672–2685.
65. Wolmark N, Wang J, et al: Preoperative chemotherapy in patients with operable breast cancer: Nine-year results from National Surgical Adjuvant Breast and Bowel Project B-18. J Natl Cancer Inst Monogr 2001; (30): 96–102.
66. Mauri D, Pavlidis N, et al: Neoadjuvant versus adjuvant systemic treatment in breast cancer: A meta-analysis. J Natl Cancer Inst 2005; 97(3): 188–194.
67. Turnbull AD, Gundy E, et al: Surgical mortality among the elderly. An analysis of 4,050 operations (1970–1974). Clin Bull 1978; 8(4): 139–142.
68. Martelli G, Miceli R, et al: Is axillary lymph node dissection necessary in elderly patients with breast carcinoma who have a clinically uninvolved axilla? Cancer 2003; 97(5): 1156–1163.
69. Hughes KS, Schnaper LA, et al: Lumpectomy plus tamoxifen with or without irradiation in women 70 years of age or older with early breast cancer. N Engl J Med 2004; 351(10): 971–977.
70. Rudenstam CM, Zahrieh D, et al: Randomized trial comparing axillary clearance versus no axillary clearance in older patients with breast cancer: First results of International Breast Cancer Study Group Trial 10-93. J Clin Oncol 2006; 24(3): 337–344.
71. Fisher B, Bryant J, et al: Tamoxifen, radiation therapy, or both for prevention of ipsilateral breast tumor recurrence after lumpectomy in women with invasive breast cancers of one centimeter or less. J Clin Oncol 2002; 20(20): 4141–4149.

72. Fentiman IS, van Zijl J, et al: Treatment of operable breast cancer in the elderly: A randomised clinical trial EORTC 10850 comparing modified radical mastectomy with tumorectomy plus tamoxifen. Eur J Cancer 2003; 39(3): 300–308.

73. Bines J, Oleske DM, et al: Ovarian function in premenopausal women treated with adjuvant chemotherapy for breast cancer. J Clin Oncol 1996; 14(5): 1718–1729.

74. Lower EE, Blau R, et al: The risk of premature menopause induced by chemotherapy for early breast cancer. J Womens Health Gend Based Med 1999; 8(7): 949–954.

75. Petrek JA, Naughton MJ, et al: Incidence, time course, and determinants of menstrual bleeding after breast cancer treatment: A prospective study. J Clin Oncol 2006; 24(7): 1045–1051.

76. Swain SM, Whaley FS, et al: Congestive heart failure in patients treated with doxorubicin: A retrospective analysis of three trials. Cancer 2003; 97(11): 2869–2879.

77. Smith RE, Bryant J, et al: Acute myeloid leukemia and myelodysplastic syndrome after doxorubicin-cyclophosphamide adjuvant therapy for operable breast cancer: The National Surgical Adjuvant Breast and Bowel Project Experience. J Clin Oncol 2003; 21(7): 1195–1204.

78. Weiss RB, Woolf SH, et al: Natural history of more than 20 years of node-positive primary breast carcinoma treated with cyclophosphamide, methotrexate, and fluorouracil-based adjuvant chemotherapy: A study by the Cancer and Leukemia Group B. J Clin Oncol 2003; 21(9): 1825–1835.

79. Robertson JF, Howell A, et al: Static disease on anastrozole provides similar benefit as objective response in patients with advanced breast cancer. Breast Cancer Res Treat 1999; 58(2): 157–162.

80. Tondini C, Hayes DF, et al: Comparison of CA15-3 and carcinoembryonic antigen in monitoring the clinical course of patients with metastatic breast cancer. Cancer Res 1988; 48(14): 4107–4112.

81. Soletormos G, Nielsen D, et al: Tumor markers cancer antigen 15.3, carcinoembryonic antigen, and tissue polypeptide antigen for monitoring metastatic breast cancer during first-line chemotherapy and follow-up. Clin Chem 1996; 42(4): 564–575.

82. Kiang DT, Greenberg LJ, et al: Tumor marker kinetics in the monitoring of breast cancer. Cancer 1990; 65(2): 193–199.

83. Stearns V, Yamauchi H, et al: Circulating tumor markers in breast cancer: Accepted utilities and novel prospects. Breast Cancer Res Treat 1998; 52(1-3): 239–259.

84. Symeonidis A, Kouraklis-Symeonidis A, et al: Increased serum CA-15.3 levels in patients with megaloblastic anemia due to vitamin B12 deficiency. Oncology 2004; 67(5-6): 359–367.

85. Fossati R, Confalonieri C, et al: Cytotoxic and hormonal treatment for metastatic breast cancer: A systematic review of published randomized trials involving 31,510 women. J Clin Oncol 1998; 16(10): 3439–3460.

86. Nabholtz JM, Buzdar A, et al: Anastrozole is superior to tamoxifen as first-line therapy for advanced breast cancer in postmenopausal women: Results of a North American multicenter randomized trial. Arimidex Study Group. J Clin Oncol 2000; 18(22): 3758–3767.

87. Mouridsen H, Gershanovich M, et al: Phase III study of letrozole versus tamoxifen as first-line therapy of advanced breast cancer in postmenopausal women: analysis of survival and update of efficacy from the International Letrozole Breast Cancer Group. J Clin Oncol 2003; 21(11): 2101–2109.

88. Forward DP, Cheung KL, et al: Clinical and endocrine data for goserelin plus anastrozole as second-line endocrine therapy for premenopausal advanced breast cancer. Br J Cancer 2004; 90(3): 590–594.

89. Plotkin D, Lechner JJ, et al: Tamoxifen flare in advanced breast cancer. JAMA 1978; 240(24): 2644–2646.

90. Howell A, Dodwell DJ, et al: Response after withdrawal of tamoxifen and progestogens in advanced breast cancer. Ann Oncol 1992; 3(8): 611–617.

91. Pyrhonen S, Ellmen J, et al: Meta-analysis of trials comparing toremifene with tamoxifen and factors predicting outcome of antiestrogen therapy in postmenopausal women with breast cancer. Breast Cancer Res Treat 1999; 56(2): 133–143.

92. Vogel CL, Shemano I, et al: Multicenter phase II efficacy trial of toremifene in tamoxifen-refractory patients with advanced breast cancer. J Clin Oncol 1993; 11(2): 345–350.

93. Buzdar AU, Jonat W, et al: Anastrozole versus megestrol acetate in the treatment of postmenopausal women with advanced breast carcinoma: Results of a survival update based on a combined analysis of data from two mature phase III trials. Arimidex Study Group. Cancer 1998; 83(6): 1142–1152.

94. Dombernowsky P, Smith I, et al: Letrozole, a new oral aromatase inhibitor for advanced breast cancer: Double-blind randomized trial showing a dose effect and improved efficacy and tolerability compared with megestrol acetate. J Clin Oncol 1998; 16(2): 453–461.

95. Kvinnsland S, Anker G, et al: High activity and tolerability demonstrated for exemestane in postmenopausal women with metastatic breast cancer who had previously failed on tamoxifen treatment. Eur J Cancer 2000; 36(8): 976–982.

96. Rose C, Vtoraya O, et al: An open randomised trial of second-line endocrine therapy in advanced breast cancer. Comparison of the aromatase inhibitors letrozole and anastrozole. Eur J Cancer 2003; 39(16): 2318–2327.

97. Lonning PE, Bajetta E, et al: Activity of exemestane in metastatic breast cancer after failure of nonsteroidal aromatase inhibitors: A phase II trial. J Clin Oncol 2000; 18(11): 2234–2244.

98. Bertelli G, Garrone O, et al: Sequential treatment with exemestane and non-steroidal aromatase inhibitors in advanced breast cancer. Oncology 2005; 69(6): 471–477.

99. Howell A, DeFriend D, et al: Response to a specific antioestrogen (ICI 182780) in tamoxifen-resistant breast cancer. Lancet 1995; 345(8941): 29–30.

100. Watanabe T, Sano M, et al: Fulvestrant for the treatment of advanced breast cancer in postmenopausal women: A Japanese study. Anticancer Res 2004; 24(2C): 1275–1280.

101. Ingle JN, Suman VJ, et al: Fulvestrant in women with advanced breast cancer after progression on prior aromatase inhibitor therapy: North Central Cancer Treatment Group Trial N0032. J Clin Oncol 2006; 24(7): 1052–1056.

102. Chan S, Friedrichs K, et al: Prospective randomized trial of docetaxel versus doxorubicin in patients with metastatic breast cancer. J Clin Oncol 1999; 17(8): 2341–2354.

103. Paridaens R, Biganzoli L, et al: Paclitaxel versus doxorubicin as first-line single-agent chemotherapy for metastatic breast cancer: A European Organization for Research and Treatment of Cancer Randomized Study with cross-over. J Clin Oncol 2000; 18(4): 724–733.

104. Jones SE, Erban J, et al: Randomized phase III study of docetaxel compared with paclitaxel in metastatic breast cancer. J Clin Oncol 2005; 23(24): 5542–5551.
105. Carrick S, Parker S, et al: Single agent versus combination chemotherapy for metastatic breast cancer. Cochrane Database Syst Rev 2005; (2): CD003372.
106. Sledge GW, Neuberg D, et al: Phase III trial of doxorubicin, paclitaxel, and the combination of doxorubicin and paclitaxel as front-line chemotherapy for metastatic breast cancer: An intergroup trial (E1193). J Clin Oncol 2003; 21(4): 588–592.
107. Conte PF, Guarneri V, et al: Concomitant versus sequential administration of epirubicin and paclitaxel as first-line therapy in metastatic breast carcinoma: results for the Gruppo Oncologico Nord Ovest randomized trial. Cancer 2004; 101(4): 704–712.
108. Farquhar C, Marjoribanks J, et al: High dose chemotherapy and autologous bone marrow or stem cell transplantation versus conventional chemotherapy for women with metastatic breast cancer. Cochrane Database Syst Rev 2005; (3): CD003142.
109. Bendell JC, Domchek SM, et al: Central nervous system metastases in women who receive trastuzumab-based therapy for metastatic breast carcinoma. Cancer 2003; 97(12): 2972–2977.
110. Clayton AJ, Danson S, et al: Incidence of cerebral metastases in patients treated with trastuzumab for metastatic breast cancer. Br J Cancer 2004; 91(4): 639–643.
111. Esteva FJ, Valero V, et al: Phase II study of weekly docetaxel and trastuzumab for patients with HER-2-overexpressing metastatic breast cancer. J Clin Oncol 2002; 20(7): 1800–1808.
112. Montemurro F, Choa G, et al: Safety and activity of docetaxel and trastuzumab in HER2 overexpressing metastatic breast cancer: A pilot phase II study. Am J Clin Oncol 2003; 26(1): 95–97.
113. Marty M, Cognetti F, et al: Randomized phase II trial of the efficacy and safety of trastuzumab combined with docetaxel in patients with human epidermal growth factor receptor 2-positive metastatic breast cancer administered as first-line treatment: The M77001 study group. J Clin Oncol 2005; 23(19): 4265–4274.
114. Perez EA, Suman VJ, et al: Two concurrent phase II trials of paclitaxel/carboplatin/trastuzumab (weekly or every-3-week schedule) as first-line therapy in women with HER2-overexpressing metastatic breast cancer: NCCTG study 983252. Clin Breast Cancer 2005; 6(5): 425–432.
115. Robert N, Leyland-Jones B, et al: Randomized phase III study of trastuzumab, paclitaxel, and carboplatin compared with trastuzumab and paclitaxel in women with HER-2-overexpressing metastatic breast cancer. J Clin Oncol 2006; 24(18): 2786–2792.
116. Burstein HJ, Kuter I, et al: Clinical activity of trastuzumab and vinorelbine in women with HER2-overexpressing metastatic breast cancer. J Clin Oncol 2001; 19(10): 2722–2730.
117. Jahanzeb M, Mortimer JE, et al: Phase II trial of weekly vinorelbine and trastuzumab as first-line therapy in patients with HER2(+) metastatic breast cancer. Oncologist 2002; 7(5): 410–417.
117a. Geyer CE, Forster J, et al: Lapatinib plus capecitabine for HER2-positive advanced breast cancer. N Engl J Med 2006; 355(26):2733–2743.
118. Burris HA 3rd, Hurwitz HI, et al: Phase I safety, pharmacokinetics, and clinical activity study of lapatinib (GW572016), a reversible dual inhibitor of epidermal growth factor receptor tyrosine kinases, in heavily pretreated patients with metastatic carcinomas. J Clin Oncol 2005; 23(23): 5305–5313.

119. Theriault RL, Lipton A, et al: Pamidronate reduces skeletal morbidity in women with advanced breast cancer and lytic bone lesions: A randomized, placebo-controlled trial. Protocol 18 Aredia Breast Cancer Study Group. J Clin Oncol 1999; 17(3): 846–854.

120. Antonelli NM, Dotters DJ, et al: Cancer in pregnancy: A review of the literature. Part I. Obstet Gynecol Surv 1996; 51(2): 125–134.

121. Smith LH, Dalrymple JL, et al: Obstetrical deliveries associated with maternal malignancy in California, 1992 through 1997. Am J Obstet Gynecol 2001; 184(7): 1504–1512; discussion 1512–1513.

122. Woo JC, Yu T, et al: Breast cancer in pregnancy: A literature review. Arch Surg 2003 138(1): 91–98; discussion 99.

123. Nagayama M, Watanabe Y, et al: Fast MR imaging in obstetrics. Radiographics 2002; 22(3): 563–580; discussion 580–582.

124. Ishida T, Yokoe T, et al: Clinicopathologic characteristics and prognosis of breast cancer patients associated with pregnancy and lactation: Analysis of case-control study in Japan. Jpn J Cancer Res 1992; 83(11): 1143–1149.

125. Zemlickis D, Lishner M, et al: Maternal and fetal outcome after breast cancer in pregnancy. Am J Obstet Gynecol 1992; 166(3): 781–787.

126. Bonnier P, Romain S, et al: Influence of pregnancy on the outcome of breast cancer: a case-control study. Société Française de Senologie et de Pathologie Mammaire Study Group. Int J Cancer 1997; 72(5): 720–727.

127. Doll DC, Ringenberg QS, et al: Antineoplastic agents and pregnancy. Semin Oncol 1989; 16(5): 337–346.

128. Berry DL, Theriault RL, et al: Management of breast cancer during pregnancy using a standardized protocol. J Clin Oncol 1999; 17(3): 855–861.

129. Isaacs RJ, Hunter W, et al: Tamoxifen as systemic treatment of advanced breast cancer during pregnancy—case report and literature review. Gynecol Oncol 2001; 80(3): 405–408.

130. Petrek JA, Dukoff R, et al: Prognosis of pregnancy-associated breast cancer. Cancer 1991; 67(4): 869–872.

131. Lethaby AE, O'Neill MA, et al: Overall survival from breast cancer in women pregnant or lactating at or after diagnosis. Auckland Breast Cancer Study Group. Int J Cancer 1996; 67(6): 751–755.

132. Giacalone PL, Laffargue F, et al: Chemotherapy for breast carcinoma during pregnancy: A French national survey. Cancer 1999; 86(11): 2266–2272.

133. Fisher B, Costantino J, et al: Lumpectomy compared with lumpectomy and radiation therapy for the treatment of intraductal breast cancer. N Engl J Med 1993; 328(22): 1581–1586.

134. Julien JP, Bijker N, et al: Radiotherapy in breast-conserving treatment for ductal carcinoma in situ: First results of the EORTC randomised phase III trial 10853. EORTC Breast Cancer Cooperative Group and EORTC Radiotherapy Group. Lancet 2000; 355(9203): 528–533.

135. Fisher B, Dignam J, et al: Tamoxifen in treatment of intraductal breast cancer: National Surgical Adjuvant Breast and Bowel Project B-24 randomised controlled trial. Lancet 1999; 353(9169): 1993–2000.

136. Houghton J, George WD, et al: Radiotherapy and tamoxifen in women with completely excised ductal carcinoma in situ of the breast in the UK, Australia, and New Zealand: Randomised controlled trial. Lancet 2003; 362(9378): 95–102.

137. Hance KW, Anderson WF, et al: Trends in inflammatory breast carcinoma incidence and survival: The surveillance, epidemiology, and end results program at the National Cancer Institute. J Natl Cancer Inst 2005; 97(13): 966–975.

138. Kleer CG, van Golen KL, et al: Molecular biology of breast cancer metastasis. Inflammatory breast cancer: Clinical syndrome and molecular determinants. Breast Cancer Res 2000; 2(6): 423–429.

139. Ellerbroek N, Holmes F, et al: Treatment of patients with isolated axillary nodal metastases from an occult primary carcinoma consistent with breast origin. Cancer 1990; 66(7): 1461–1467.

140. Merson M, Andreola S, et al: Breast carcinoma presenting as axillary metastases without evidence of a primary tumor. Cancer 1992; 70(2): 504–508.

141. Foroudi F. Tiver KW: Occult breast carcinoma presenting as axillary metastases. Int J Radiat Oncol Biol Phys 2000; 47(1): 143–147.

142. Cutuli B, Lacroze M, et al: Male breast cancer: Results of the treatments and prognostic factors in 397 cases. Eur J Cancer 1995; 31A(12): 1960–1964.

143. Giordano SH, Cohen DS, et al: Breast carcinoma in men: A population-based study. Cancer 2004; 101(1): 51–57.

144. Ottini L, Masala G, et al: BRCA1 and BRCA2 mutation status and tumor characteristics in male breast cancer: A population-based study in Italy. Cancer Res 2003; 63(2): 342–347.

145. Liede A, Karlan BY, et al: Cancer risks for male carriers of germline mutations in BRCA1 or BRCA2: A review of the literature. J Clin Oncol 2004; 22(4): 735–742.

146. Donegan WL, Redlich PN, et al: Carcinoma of the breast in males: A multiinstitutional survey. Cancer 1998; 83(3): 498–509.

147. Giordano SH, Valero V, et al: Efficacy of anastrozole in male breast cancer. Am J Clin Oncol 2002; 25(3): 235–237.

148. Zabolotny BP, Zalai CV, et al: Successful use of letrozole in male breast cancer: A case report and review of hormonal therapy for male breast cancer. J Surg Oncol 2005; 90(1): 26–30.

149. Kamby C. The pattern of metastases in human breast cancer: methodological aspects and influence of prognostic factors. Cancer Treat Rev 1990; 17(1): 37–61.

150. Schouten LJ, Rutten J, et al: Incidence of brain metastases in a cohort of patients with carcinoma of the breast, colon, kidney, and lung and melanoma. Cancer 2002; 94(10): 2698–2705.

151. Miller KD, Weathers T, et al: Occult central nervous system involvement in patients with metastatic breast cancer: Prevalence, predictive factors and impact on overall survival. Ann Oncol 2003; 14(7): 1072–1077.

152. Glantz MJ, Cole BF, et al: Practice parameter: Anticonvulsant prophylaxis in patients with newly diagnosed brain tumors. Report of the Quality Standards Subcommittee of the American Academy of Neurology. Neurology 2000; 54(10): 1886–1893.

153. Forsyth PA, Weaver S, et al: Prophylactic anticonvulsants in patients with brain tumour. Can J Neurol Sci 2003; 30(2): 106–112.

154. Sorensen S, Borgesen SE, et al: Metastatic epidural spinal cord compression. Results of treatment and survival. Cancer 1990; 65(7): 1502–1508.

155. Maranzano E, Latini P, et al: Radiation therapy in metastatic spinal cord compression. A prospective analysis of 105 consecutive patients. Cancer 1991; 67(5): 1311–1317.

156. Hill ME, Richards MA, et al: Spinal cord compression in breast cancer: A review of 70 cases. Br J Cancer 1993; 68(5): 969–973.

157. Helweg-Larsen S. Clinical outcome in metastatic spinal cord compression. A prospective study of 153 patients. Acta Neurol Scand 1996; 94(4): 269–275.

158. Patchell RA, Tibbs PA, et al: Direct decompressive surgical resection in the treatment of spinal cord compression caused by metastatic cancer: A randomised trial. Lancet 2005; 366(9486): 643–648.

159. Chamberlain MC, Sandy AD, et al: Leptomeningeal metastasis: A comparison of gadolinium-enhanced MR and contrast-enhanced CT of the brain. Neurology 1990; 40(3 Pt 1): 435–438.

160. Freilich RJ, Krol G, et al: Neuroimaging and cerebrospinal fluid cytology in the diagnosis of leptomeningeal metastasis. Ann Neurol 1995; 38(1): 51–57.

161. Wasserstrom WR, Glass JP, et al: Diagnosis and treatment of leptomeningeal metastases from solid tumors: Experience with 90 patients. Cancer 1982; 49(4): 759–772.

162. Grossman SA, Finkelstein DM, et al: Randomized prospective comparison of intraventricular methotrexate and thiotepa in patients with previously untreated neoplastic meningitis. Eastern Cooperative Oncology Group. J Clin Oncol 1993; 11(3): 561–569.

163. Fizazi K, Asselain B, et al: Meningeal carcinomatosis in patients with breast carcinoma. Clinical features, prognostic factors, and results of a high-dose intrathecal methotrexate regimen. Cancer 1996; 77(7): 1315–1323.

164. Jaeckle KA, Phuphanich S, et al: Intrathecal treatment of neoplastic meningitis due to breast cancer with a slow-release formulation of cytarabine. Br J Cancer 2001; 84(2): 157–163.

165. Goldhirsch A, Glick JH, et al: Meeting highlights: International expert consensus on the primary therapy of early breast cancer 2005. Ann Oncol 2005; 16(10): 1569–1583.

166. NCCN guidelines available from http://www.nccn.org/professionals/physician_gls/PDF/breast.pdf [accessed 25 September 2006].

FIGURE CREDITS

The following book published by Gower Medical Publishing is a source of figures in the present chapter. The figure numbers given in the listing are those of the figures in the present chapter. The page numbers given in parentheses are those of the original publication.

Hayes DF, ed: Atlas of Breast Cancer. Mosby Europe, London, 1993: Figs 4.1 (p. 1.3); 4.2 (p. 1.3); 4.3 (p. 5.5); 4.7 (p. 5.14); 4.8 (p. 5.14); 4.9 (p. 5.12); 4.10 (p. 5.12); 4.11 (p. 5.17).

Systemic and mucocutaneous reactions to chemotherapy

5

Joseph P. Eder and Arthur T. Skarin

Cancer chemotherapy is a major component of cancer therapy, along with surgery and radiation. Cancer chemotherapy agents differ from most drugs in that it is intentionally cytotoxic to human cells. This aspect of cancer chemotherapeutic agents produces a narrow therapeutic index (desired vs. undesired effects) for most, but not all, agents in this class. The target of cancer chemotherapeutic agents is the proliferating cancer cell. While many normal tissues are non-proliferating, some are proliferating and toxicity of this class tends to preferentially overlap proliferating tissues – haematopoietic, gastrointestinal mucosa and skin. In addition, each agent often has specific organ toxicity related to its chemical class or unique mechanism of action.

The major groups of cancer chemotherapeutic agents are the direct-acting alkylating agents, the indirect-acting anthracyclines and topoisomerase inhibitors, the antimetabolites, the tubulin-binding agents, hormones, receptor-targeted agents and a class of miscellaneous agents. Despite the disparate nature of this broad class of agents, some generalizations about the effects of chemotherapy are still possible. For more information readers are referred to detailed reports.[1,2]

ACUTE HYPERSENSITIVITY REACTIONS

Acute hypersensitivity can occur with any drug. However, several cancer chemotherapeutic agents are derived from hydrophobic plant chemicals and must be solubilized with agents with a marked propensity for causing acute hypersensitivity reactions, especially histamine-mediated anaphylactic reactions, such as the Cremophor used with paclitaxel. Docetaxel has a lower incidence of this complication.

The incidence of severe hypersensitivity reactions with paclitaxel may be up to 25% without ancillary measures. With antihistamine H1 and H2 blockade and corticosteroids, the incidence falls to 2–3%. Hypersensitivity reactions occur in up to 40% of patients receiving single agent 1-asparaginase but only 20% when administered in combination therapy with glucocorticoids and 6-mercaptopurine, perhaps as a result of immunosuppression. The hypersensitivity usually occurs after several doses and in successive cycles. The reaction may be only urticaria (see Figure 5.1) but may be severe with laryngospasm or, rarely, serum sickness. Fatal reactions occur <1% of the time. Changing the source of enzyme is the appropriate initial step. Two other proteins in

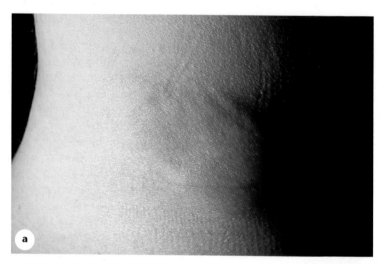

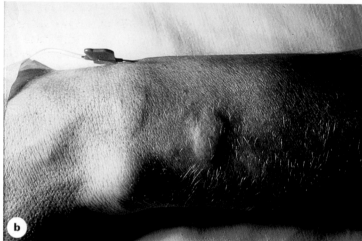

Fig. 5.1 Acute hypersensitivity reactions. Urticaria, with giant localized hives, occurred (**a**) in a 40-year-old man within a few minutes of receiving intravenous 5-fluorouracil and (**b**) in the lower arm of a 50-year-old man after receiving adriamycin. The urticaria was self-limiting in both patients.

clinical use, rituximab and traztuzumab, have a similar incidence of hypersensitivity reactions.

Certain drugs such as etoposide are associated with a greater incidence of reactions but most are not true hypersensitivity reactions. The Tween diluant in the clinical etoposide formulation produces hypotension, rash and back pain. The platinum compounds carboplatin and cisplatin are associated with hypersensitivity reactions, particularly on subsequent cycles – most of these reactions are severe (75%).[3] Hypersensitivity to platinum and related compounds is actually quite frequent, up to 14% in industrial workers, so such reactions in patients receiving these agents parenterally should not be surprising and is often unappreciated in combination chemotherapy regimens, such as with taxanes, and may be equally suppressed by the prophylactic regimens employed.[4] Liposomal encapsulated anthracyclines are associated with an increased incidence of hypersensitivity compared with the parent drugs. Like the reaction to Cremophor EL and radiocontrast agents, the reaction is a "complement activation pseudoallergy".[5] Up to 45% of cancer patients show activation of the classical, alternative or both complement pathways, although the incidence of clinical reactions is about 20%.

Monoclonal antibodies such as trastuzumab, rituximab, bevacizumab, and cetuximab have had enormous impact on cancer therapeutics. Monoclonal antibodies may be chimeric (a murine Fab binding site but human amino acid sequences elsewhere) or fully human. Allergic or hypersensitivity reactions are more frequent with chimeric proteins such as cetuximab (1–5% clinically significant) and are treated with antihistamines and steroids plus slowing of the infusion. L-Asparaginase is a bacterial protein that frequently results in hypersensitivity reactions. These reactions are more frequent with interrupted schedules and with subsequent re-challenge. Changing the source from *Escherichia coli* to *Erwinia* is one accepted strategem if immunosuppression does not work.

ALOPECIA

Many antineoplastic drugs can produce marked hair loss (see Figure 5.2). This includes not only scalp hair but also facial, axillary, pubic and all body hair. The germinating hair follicle has an approximately 24-hour doubling time. Cancer chemotherapy agents preferentially affect actively growing (anagen) hairs. The interruption of mitosis produces a structurally weakened hair prone to fracture easily from minimal trauma such as brushing. Since 80–90% of scalp hairs are in anagen phase, the degree

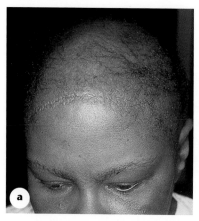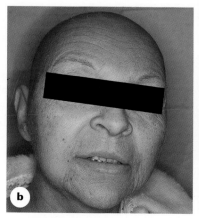

Fig. 5.2 Alopecia. (**a**) Near-total alopecia in a 38-year-old woman receiving cyclophosphamide and adriamycin. Note the loss of eyebrow and eyelid hair. (**b**) Total alopecia developed in this 64-year-old woman due to chemotherapy and cranial irradiation for brain metastases. The duration of alopecia after both treatment modalities may be many months or even permanent in some patients. In this woman, the scalp oedema and erythema are related to an allergic cutaneous reaction from diphenyl hydantoin.

of hair loss can be substantial. Hair loss, while often emotionally difficult for patients, is reversible, although hair may regrow more curly and of a slightly different colour.

STOMATITIS/MUCOSITIS

The oral complications of cancer chemotherapy are many and frequently severe. The disruption of the protective mucosal barrier serves as a portal of entry for pathogens which, especially when combined with chemotherapy-induced neutropenia, predisposes to local infection and systemic sepsis. Once established, these infections may be difficult to eradicate in immunocompromised patients. The most common infectious organisms are *Candida albicans*, herpes simplex virus, β-haemolytic streptococci, staphylococci, opportunistic Gram-negative bacteria and mouth anaerobes.

Several agents of the antimetabolite class of cancer chemotherapeutic agents, especially those that target pyrimidine biosynthesis such as methotrexate, 5-fluorouracil (5-FU) and cytosine arabinoside, and the anthracyline agents, such as doxorubicin and daunorubicin, are particularly toxic to the mucosal epithelium (see Figure 5.3). These agents

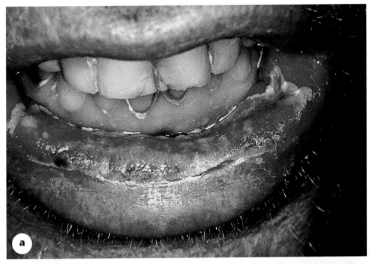

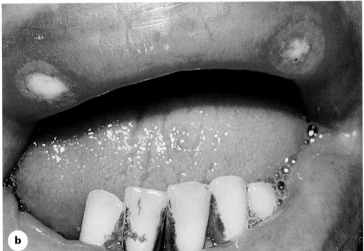

Fig. 5.3 Stomatitis and mucositis. (**a**) Marked stomatitis in a patient receiving methotrexate. (**b**) Aphthous stomatitis related to severe granulocytopenia after chemotherapy. The ulcers may be due to herpes simplex or other infection.

have a marked capacity to produce more severe injury in irradiated tissues, even if the radiation is temporally remote. These agents produce marked ulceration and erosion of the mucosa. These lesions occur initially on those mucosal surfaces that abrade the teeth and gums, such as the sides of the tongue, the vermillion border of the lower lip and the

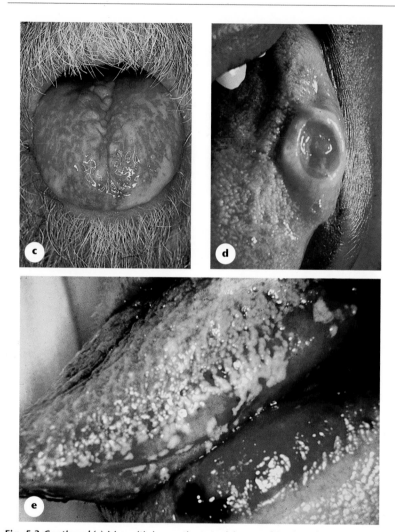

Fig. 5.3 *Continued* (**c**) Mucositis in a patient receiving combination chemotherapy for head and neck cancer. (**d**) Marked ulcer of the tongue in a 32-year-old man receiving induction chemotherapy for acute leukaemia. (**e**) Mucositis of the tongue due to monilia infection (thrush) in a patient receiving corticosteroids for brain metastases.

buccal mucosa. More advanced mucosal injury may occur on the hard and soft palate and the posterior oropharynx. These ulcerations cannot often be distinguished from those caused by infectious organisms. Appropriate tests must be performed to exclude viral, fungal and bacterial causes or superinfection.

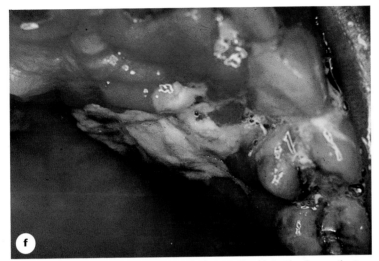

Fig. 5.3 *Continued* (f) Marked oral mucositis due to mixed infection in a patient receiving chemotherapy for acute leukaemia.

In addition to the risk of infection, the resultant pain makes patients unable to maintain adequate nutrition and hydration. This may compromise the capacity to complete a course of chemotherapy and require prolonged administration of parenteral fluids and even parenteral nutrition.

DERMATITIS, SKIN RASHES AND HYPERPIGMENTATION

Superficial manifestations of cancer chemotherapy agents are noted frequently by patients, although they are considered significant much less often by clinicians. The cosmetic changes may be disturbing to patients without requiring discontinuation of therapy.

Of the direct-acting alkylating agents, busulfan has been associated with a wide variety of specific and non-specific cutaneous changes. Diffuse hyperpigmentation has been noted (see Figure 5.4), which resolves with discontinuation of therapy. Systemic mechlorethamine (nitrogen mustard) has no cutaneous toxicity. However, when applied topically for cutaneous T-cell lymphomas, telangiectasias, hyperpigmentation and allergic contact dermatitis may occur. The development of more effective, safer alternative agents has rendered busulfan and mechlorethamine to essentially historical interest only or narrow

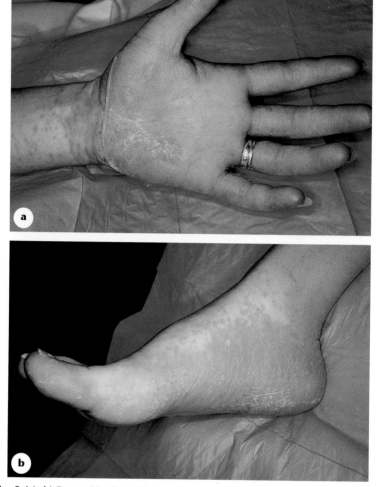

Fig. 5.4 (a,b) Dermatitis, skin rashes and hyperpigmentation: hand–foot syndrome related to 5-fluorouracil chemotherapy in metastatic colon cancer. Note the erythema, oedema, rash and early skin desquamation. Severe pain is associated with this toxic reaction.

indications (busulfan in allogeneic bone marrow transplant for haematological malignancies). Cyclophosphamide, ifosfamide and melphalan produce hyperpigmentation of nails, teeth, gingiva and skin.

The antimetabolites methotrexate and 5-FU are frequently associated with cutaneous reactions. In contrast, the purine antimetabolites

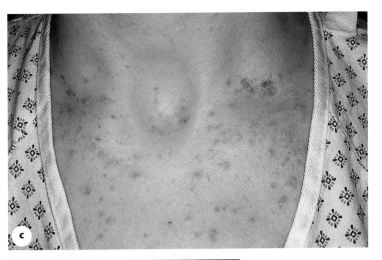

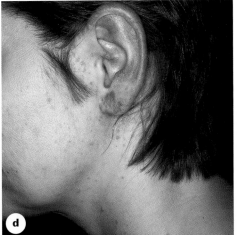

Fig. 5.4 *Continued* (**c,d**) Skin reaction to Ara-C. Note the erythematous macular rash on the chest and diffuse erythema and oedema of the ears in this 22-year-old woman receiving Ara-C for acute leukaemia.

6-mercaptopurine, 6-thioguanine, cladribine, fludarabine and pento-statin are devoid of cutaneous toxicity. Methotrexate, a folate antago-nist, may cause reactivation of ultraviolet burns when given in close proximity to previous sun exposure. This is not prevented by leucov-orin, a reduced folate that prevents the myelosuppression and stom-

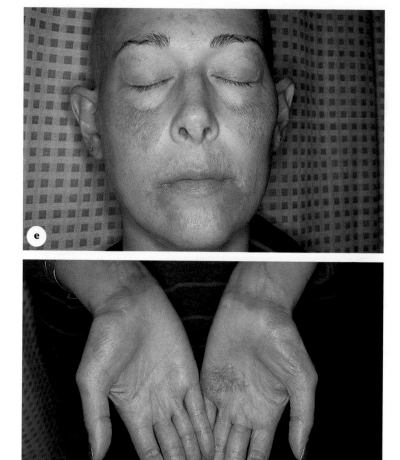

Fig. 5.4 *Continued* (e,f) Skin reaction to docetaxel. Note periorbital and malar flush along with erythema and oedema of the palms in this patient.

atitis of high doses of methotrexate. Methotrexate should be given more than a week after a significant solar burn. It may cause stomatitis and cutaneous ulcerations at high dose, despite the use of leucovorin. Extensive epidermal necrolysis may occur and be fatal. Multiple areas of vesiculation and erosion over pressure areas have been noticed.

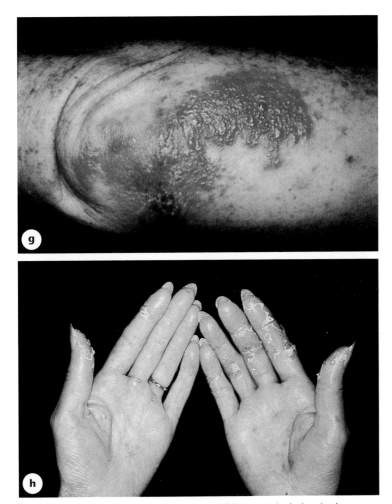

Fig. 5.4 *Continued* (**g,h**) Cutaneous reactions to bleomycin include raised, erythematous and pruritic lesions around pressure points, especially the elbows (**g**), as well as desquamation of skin (**h**).

5-FU is an antimetabolite with steric properties similar to uracil. Like methotrexate, 5-FU produces increased sensitivity to ultraviolet-induced toxic reactions in a large number of patients, over 35% in one study. Enhanced sunburn erythema and increased posterythema hyper-pigmentation characterize these reactions. A hyperpigmentation reaction over the veins in which the drug is administered may occur. This is

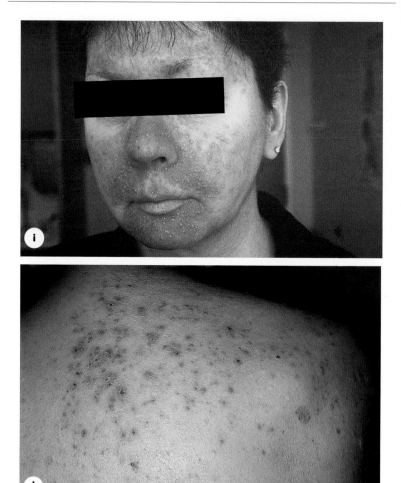

Fig. 5.4 *Continued* (**i,j**) Acneiform skin lesions occur in patients on gefitinib, especially on the face (**i**), chest and back (**j**). These rashes may regress when the drug is temporarily withheld or the dose is lowered. Similar skin reactions occur after actinomycin D and corticosteroids.

probably hyperpigmentation secondary to chemical phlebitis due to chemotherapeutic agents in the superficial venous system. Nail and generalized skin hyperpigmentation have been reported with 5-FU. Occasionally, acute inflammation of existing actinic keratosis is seen in patients receiving 5-FU. This differs from a drug reaction in that it occurs in discrete inflamed regions only in sun-exposed areas, not in a

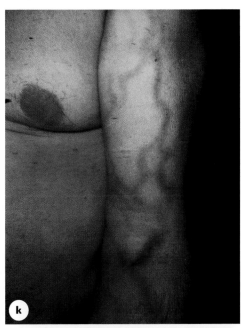

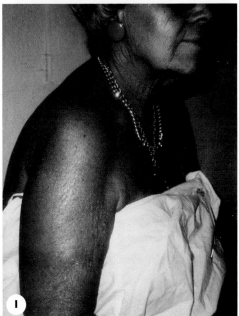

Fig. 5.4 *Continued* **(k)** Hyperpigmentation of the skin along veins occurs after the use of many chemotherapeutic agents, including Navelbine, actinomycin D and 5-fluorouracil infusion, as in this patient. In many cases, the veins become sclerotic due to thrombophlebitis. **(l–n)** Hyperpigmentation of the skin after 5-fluorouracil **(l)**, *Continued*

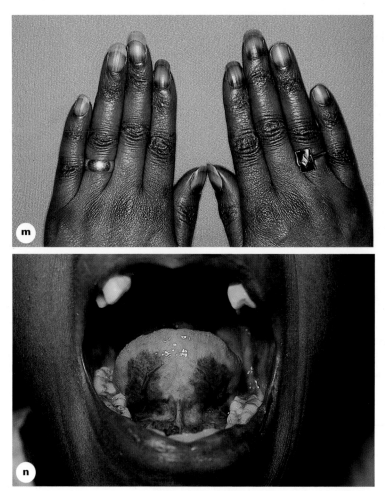

Fig. 5.4 *Continued* Hyperpigmentation of the skin occurs after adriamycin and other drugs (**m**), while increased pigment in the mucous membranes (**n**) and nails (**m**) is mainly related to adriamycin. (Also see Fig. 5.6b).

generalized distribution. The end result is usually the disappearance of the actinic keratosis as a result of an inflammatory infiltration into the atypical epidermis and resultant removal of atypical cells.

When 5-FU is given by intravenous continuous infusion, the most common dose-limiting toxicity is erythromalagia, the so-called hand–foot syndrome (see Figure 5.4). The hands and feet become red, oedematous and often painful. The skin often peels afterwards. The nails become dry and brittle and develop linear cracks. This may occur at doses less than those that produce the hand–foot syndrome. Other drugs that can result in this syndrome include new, targeted therapy drugs, such as sorafenib and sunitinib, which have multiple targets including vascular endothelial growth factor (VEGF) receptor. A similar reaction occurs with 5-FU or 5-FU prodrugs administered orally on a daily schedule. Capecitabine, an oral prodrug that is eventually converted to 5-FU intracellularly, produces erythromalagia as its most common toxicity. Interestingly, oral 5-FU does not produce this syndrome when combined with enyluracil, an irreversible inhibitor of dihydropyrimidine dehydrogenase, the major enzyme in 5-FU catabolism.

High doses of cytosine arabinoside may produce ocular toxicity through an ulcerating keratoconjunctivitis. This may be prevented by the prophylactic administration of steroid eyedrops. Excessive lacrimation may be noted with 5-FU therapy due to lacrimal duct stenosis. This is corrected by surgical dilatation of the duct.

The indirect acting anticancer drugs may produce superficial cutaneous toxicity. The anthracyclines doxorubicin, daunorubicin, epirubicin and idarubicin produce complete alopecia. Radiation recall reactions are frequent, even when the two modalities are separated by years. Skin, nail and mucous membrane hyperpigmentation may be striking; these may be localized or general. Hyperpigmentation of the hands, feet and face may occur in patients of African descent. Liposomal anthracyclines, such as Doxil (doxorubicin) and Daunosome (daunorubicin), may produce a severe erythromayalagia with palmar and plantar erythema and desquamation similar to 5-FU. Actinomycin D produces a characteristic skin eruption in many patients. Beginning 3–5 days after drug administration, patients develop facial erythema followed by papules, pustules and plugged follicles similar to the open comedones of acne. This eruption is benign, self-limited and not a reason to stop therapy. A similar acneiform skin rash occurs in patients taking the new oral epidermal growth factor receptor inhibitors such as gefitinib and erlotinib (see Figure 5.4). In most patients the rash is mild and may regress with continued treatment. When severe, the skin lesions will rapidly regress with discontinuation of the drug. Topical steroids and antibiotics may be indicated.

Bleomycin is actually a mixture of peptides isolated from *Streptomyces verticullus*. Its most common toxic effects involve the lungs and skin because of high concentrations in these organs due to the deficiency of the catabolic enzyme bleomycin hydrolase in these tissues. Cutaneous toxicity occurs in the majority of patients treated with bleomycin doses in excess of 200 mg. Bleomycin causes a morbilliform eruption 30 minutes to 3 hours after administration in approximately 10% of patients (see Figure 5.4). It most likely represents a transient hypersensitivity response (it may be accompanied by fever). Linear or "flagellate" hyperpigmentation may occur on the trunk. This may likewise represent postinflammatory hyperpigmentation. Bleomycin may cause a scleroderma-like eruption of the skin. Infiltrative plaques, nodules and linear bands of the hands have been described. Pathological findings include dermal sclerosis and appendage entrapment similar to that seen in scleroderma. These changes are reversible when the drug is stopped.

Etoposide has relatively few cutaneous manifestations at standard doses (<600 mg/m^2). At higher doses (1800–4200 mg/m^2), a generalized pruritic, erythematous, maculopapular rash occurs in approximately 25% of patients. The most severe toxicity occurs at the highest doses. In these patients, an intense, well-defined palmar erythema develops. Affected areas become oedematous, red and painful. Bullus formation and desquamation follow. The severity of the reaction is related to dose. A short course (3–5 days) of corticosteroids controls the symptoms.

Sorafenib and a related drug, sunitinib malate, are oral multi-targeted receptor tyrosine kinase inhibitors that block signal transduction through the *raf* kinases, vascular endothelial growth factor receptor 2 (VEGFR2) and the platelet-derived growth factor receptors. At the recommended dose there is a 33% incidence of skin rashes or desquamation, 27% incidence of hand–foot syndome and 22% incidence of alopecia (all grades of severity).[6]

Cutaneous rashes are the most common toxicities encountered with gefitinib and erlotinib. The chimeric monoclonal antibodies cetuximab and panitumumab are associated with dermatological toxicity. The severity and extent of the skin changes, including dry skin, desquamation, erythema, nail changes and acneiform eruptions varies from report to report and no consistent grading system for incidence and severity is universally agreed upon. There is neutrophil and macrophage infiltration of the dermis and hair follicles, with thinning of the epidermis and stratum corneum. The incidence and severity is dose-dependent. Certain epidermal growth factor receptor polymorphisms increase the incidence of developing a rash. For erlotinib, cetuximab and panitumumab, several studies support a positive correlation between development of a rash and response, and rash and survival.[7] Management is usually supportive with creams, including 1% clindamycin, 5% benzoyl peroxide and systemic antibiotics when there is evidence of infection, including tetracycline and amoxicillin/clavulinate. These should be used only when necessary.

SKIN ULCERATION AND EXTRAVASATION

Vesicant reactions from extravasated cancer chemotherapeutic agents are one of the most debilitating complications seen with cancer therapy (see Figure 5.5). The anthracyclines, especially doxorubicin, are particularly noted for an intense inflammatory chemical cellulitis caused by

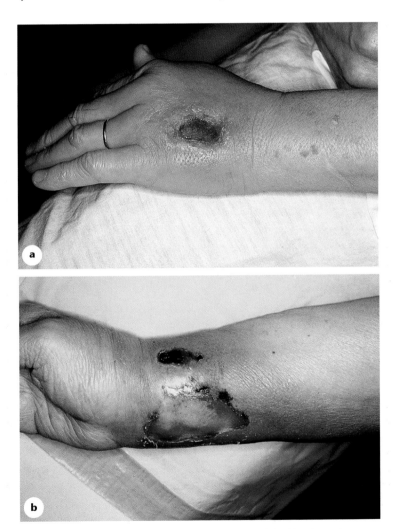

Fig. 5.5 (a–d) Extravasation of drugs and skin ulcers occurs with vesicant drugs. Acute changes with adriamycin (**a,b**)

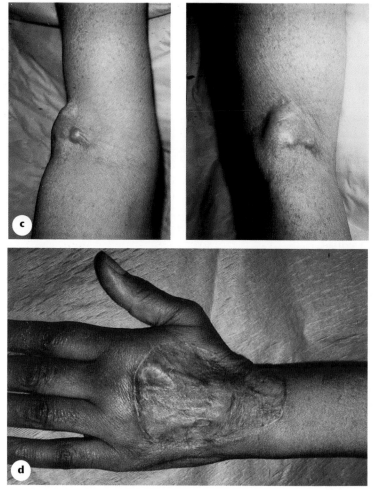

Fig. 5.5 Continued (**c**) Chronic healed scarring with adriamycin, (**d**) mitomycin-C. Other drugs include actinomycin D, vincristine and Navelbine. Immediate medical attention is necessary and sometimes skin grafts are required (see text).

subcutaneous extravasation. This results in ulceration and necrosis of affected tissue. No local measures have proven unequivocally helpful once the accident has occurred. Doxorubicin should be stopped immediately but the intravenous line left in place. Dilution of doxorubicin with sodium bicarbonate and the local installation of steroids prior to catheter withdrawal are standard measures but their efficacy is uncertain. Rest and warm compresses are recommended. If healing does not proceed well, excision of the affected area and surgical grafting are recommended to avoid excess morbidity. Other agents with vesicant properties include the vinca alkaloids (vincristine, vinblastine, vinorelbine) and actinomycin. General recommendations for the administration of vesicant drugs include the use of veins as far away from the hands and joints as possible and that the intravenous line be able to infuse at a rapid rate and have a good blood return. The use of venous access devices is accepted as appropriate in this situation unless contraindicated on specific clinical grounds.

Generalized skin ulceration is an infrequent, albeit dramatic, occurrence. Mucocutaneous ulcerations are frequently noted with bleomycin. These begin as oedema and erythema over pressure points such as the elbows, knees and fingertips and in intertrigenous areas such as the groin and axillae. These areas then proceed to shallow ulcerations. These ulcerations may also occur in the oral cavity. Biopsy shows epidermal degeneration and necrosis with dermal oedema. Total epidermal necrosis can even be found without any dermal changes. This suggests that the epidermal toxicity is the primary event.

NAIL CHANGES

Banding of the nails is the appearance of linear horizontal depressions in the nails that occur as a result of growth interruptions in the nail germinal cell layer by a cytostatic effect from the administration of cancer chemotherapy agents. These occur in other disease settings and are called Beau's lines (see Figure 5.6). The direct-acting alkylating agents cyclophosphamide, ifosfamide and melphalan may also produce hyperpigmentation of nails. The nails may exhibit linear or transverse banding or hyperpigmentation. These changes begin proximally and progress distally and clear, proximally to distally, when the agents are discontinued. Similar effects are seen with the indirect–acting anthracyclines, such as doxorubicin, and bleomycin. The anthracyclines may cause hyperpigmentation of the hyponychia (the soft layer of skin beneath the nail), especially in dark-skinned persons.

Onycholysis is separation of the nail plate from the nail bed (see Figure 5.6). Anthracyclines, anthracenediones and taxanes are the drugs most frequently associated with onycholysis. The combination of these agents is most frequently reported with onycholysis. Most of the reports are associated with docetaxel, either administered weekly or every 3

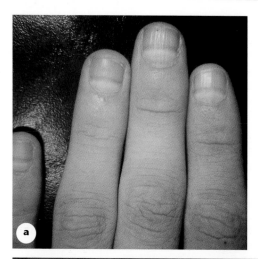

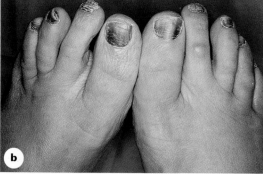

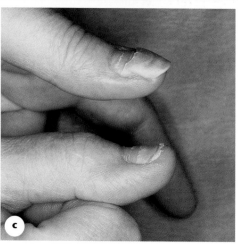

Fig. 5.6 Nail changes are often seen after prolonged chemotherapy. (**a**) Banding of the nails results from growth interruptions in the nail germinal cell layer by the cytostatic effect of chemotherapy. These white bands (called Mee's lines) will grow outward eventually. Beau's lines are transverse grooves across the nail plate due to temporary nail matrix malfunction, seen with chemotherapy or associated with other illnesses (acute coronary or severe febrile episodes). Nail hyperpigmentation occurs occasionally after prolonged use of adriamycin (**b**) especially in people with dark skin. Onycholysis or separation of the nail from its bed is associated with use of adriamycin (**c**), cyclophosphamide and the taxanes.

weeks. These changes occur after hyperpigmentation of the hyponychia, often with hyperkeratosis and splinter haemorrhages. Ultraviolet light may be a facilitating factor. Onycholysis can occur within weeks or months of the initiation of therapy.

RADIATION RECALL

Radiation recall dermatitis is a cutaneous toxicity that develops in patients with prior exposure to therapeutic doses of radiation and subsequent treatment with a cancer chemotherapeutic agent (see Figure 5.7). These reactions occur in the previously irradiated field and not elsewhere. A previous cutaneous reaction at the time of irradiation is not a prerequisite. The onset of symptoms is days to weeks after drug treatment and can occur any time after radiation, even years later. Cutaneous manifestations include erythema with maculopapular eruptions, vesiculation and desquamation. The intensity of the cutaneous response can vary from a mild rash to skin necrosis. Radiation recall reactions in other organs can produce gastrointestinal mucosal inflammation (stomatitis, oesophagitis, enteritis, proctitis), pneumonitis and myocarditis.

An extensive number of anticancer agents have been implicated in radiation recall reactions. The anthracyclines (doxorubicin as an example), bleomycin, dactinomycin, etoposide, the taxanes, vinca alkaloids and antimetabolites (hydroxycarbamide, fluorouracil, methotrexate, gemcitabine) are the most commonly implicated in cutaneous toxicity. In addition, these skin reactions have been seen in association with targeted therapy with drugs such as gefitinib.

Methotrexate and dactinomycin are reported to cause radiation enhancement in the central nervous system (CNS). The antimetabolites doxorubicin, dactinomycin and bleomycin enhance gastrointestinal toxicity from radiation. Cyclophosphamide, taxanes, hydroxycarbamide, doxorubicin, dactinomycin, gemcitabine, cytosine arabinoside and, most importantly, bleomycin exacerbate pulmonary radiation toxicity. Optic toxicity is increased by treatment with fluorouracil and cytosine arabinoside. Radiation lowers the dose of doxorubicin that produces cardiomyopathy.

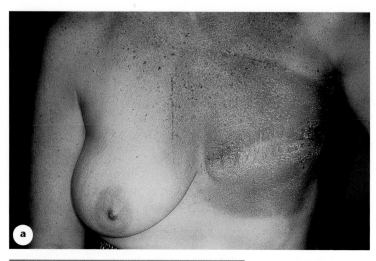

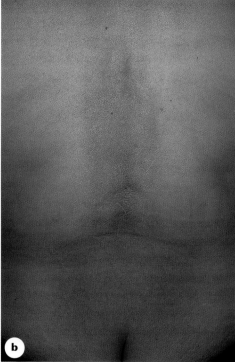

Fig. 5.7 Radiation recall dermatitis may occur in a radiotherapy treatment field after systemic chemotherapy, with development of hyperaemia and then hyperpigmentation in the healing phase (**a**). The patient in (**a**) received adjuvant Alkeran (melphalan) 1 month after postoperative radiation to the chest wall. (**b**) This patient had radiation therapy to the lower spine for bone metastases from breast cancer and developed recall dermatitis 6 months later, when gemcitabine was administered.

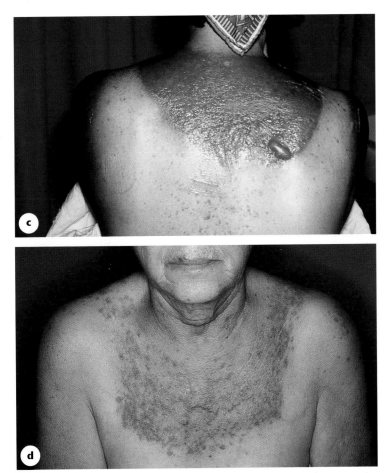

Fig. 5.7 *Continued* (**c**) Chemotherapy can also sensitize the skin to adverse reactions to solar radiation. This young woman developed severe dermatitis in a sun-exposed area while taking methotrexate. (**d**) This patient also developed acute dermatitis in a sun-exposed area while receiving 5-fluorouracil.

ORGAN TOXICITY

CARDIAC AND CARDIOVASCULAR TOXICITY

Cardiotoxicity is a well-recognized consequence of anthracycline use, especially doxorubicin because of its wide spectrum of antineoplastic therapy. This peculiar and potentially lethal problem can be classified as acute or chronic. The acute toxicity is usually asymptomatic arrhythmias, including heart block. Acute myopericarditis occurs at low total doses in an idiosyncratic fashion or at high single doses >110–120 mg/m^2. Fever, pericarditis and congestive heart failure (CHF) are the clinical manifestations. Chronic cardiomyopathy is characterized by progressive myofibrillar damage with each dose, dilatation of sarcoplasmic reticulum, loss of myofibrils and myocardial necrosis/fibrosis. Various syndromes of cardiac toxicity related to antineoplastic agents have been recently reviewed in detail.[8] Imatinib mesylate used commonly in chronic myelogenous leukaemia and gastrointestinal stromal tumours, has been associated with a low incidence of cardiomyopathy syndrome.[9]

A doxorubicin total dose <550 mg/m^2 has a 1–10% occurrence of CHF (daunorubicin 900–1000 mg/m^2), a 40% incidence at 800 mg/m^2 of doxorubicin, and the incidence of CHF approaches 100% at 1 g/m^2. Cardiac function is tested using non-invasive techniques to measure the resting and exercise ejection fraction, including radionuclide ventriculograms and echocardiograms, or invasively by cardiac biopsy. Factors that increase the risk of developing CHF include pre-existing heart disease, hypertension and cardiac radiation therapy. Concomitant dosing with trastuzamab increases the cardiac toxicity of doxorubicin. Cardiac toxicity is a function of *peak* dose level, so continuous infusions or weekly dosing decrease the risk. Desrazoxane, an iron chelator, decreases cardiotoxicity and is approved for use.

Biochemical mechanisms implicated include calcium-mediated damage to the sarcoplasmic reticulum which increases calcium ion (Ca^{++}) release with increased Ca^{++} uptake in mitochondria in preference to ATP. Lipid peroxidations of the sarcoplasmic reticulum, which decrease high Ca^{++} binding sites, and lipid peroxidation due to drug $\cdot$Fe^{3+} complexes with hydroxyl (OH) radical generation may contribute to cardiotoxicity. The heart has no catalase, and anthracyclines decrease glutathione peroxidase activity, which increases the sensitivity of the myocardium to oxidative damage.

Idarubicin and epirubicin have less cardiotoxicity but are still capable of causing cardiotoxicity. High-dose cyclophosphamide, at doses

>60 mg/kg as used in bone marrow transplantation, can cause a haemor-rhagic cardiomyopathy. Paclitaxel produces clinically insignificant atrial arrhythmias. Agents that can produce arterial smooth muscle spasm may produce ischaemic myocardial infarction in the absence of fixed coronary vascular disease. These agents include 5-FU, vincristine and vinblastine.

Combination chemotherapy in colorectal cancer with bevacizumab has been associated with an incidence (1–3%) of ischaemic cardiac events above that observed with conventional therapy alone. This increase in cardiovascular events, while of low overall incidence, nonetheless represents about a 3-fold increase.[10]

Sunitinib has a 10% incidence of usually reversible cardiomyopathy. Patients can often be treated with lower doses if and when symptoms resolve.[11]

Hypertension has been recognized as a class effect for agents that target VEGFR2. Hypertension is so common that it serves as a pharmacodynamic endpoint in the early development of agents of this class. Hypertension of a moderate degree (grade 2, recurrent or persistent, symptomatic increase of diastolic blood pressure >200 mmHg or to >150/100 mmHg or requiring monotherapy) or severe degree (grade 3, requiring more than one agent or more intensive therapy) occurs in 10–25% of patients receiving bevacizumab, sorafenib or sunitinib. Patients with pre-existing or borderline hypertension are more susceptible. No specific treatment algorithmn has yet been applied to the management of these patients.

PULMONARY TOXICITY

Bleomycin produces pulmonary toxicity, which is the major problem with subacute or chronic interstitial pneumonitis complicated by late-stage fibrosis (see Figure 5.8). The incidence is 3–5% with doses <450 u/m^2, in patients over 70, with emphysema and after high single doses (>25 u/m^2). The incidence rises to 10% at doses >450 mg/m^2, but can occur at cumulative doses <100 mg. Pulmonary injury can occur during high FiO$_2$ and volume overload during surgery for many years after exposure.

Toxicity results from free radicals produced by an intercalated Fe(II)–bleomycin–O$_2$ complex between DNA strands. Intercalation of drug into the DNA is the first step; then Fe(II) is oxidized and O$_2$ is reduced to oxygen ($^{\bullet}$O$_2$) or hydroxyl radicals $^{\bullet}$OH. DNA cleavage occurs after the activated bleomycin complex is assembled. Strand breakage absolutely requires O$_2$, which is converted to O$_2$ and $^{\bullet}$OH, and peroxidation products of DNA (and protein) are formed. Free radical scavengers and superoxide dismutase inhibit DNA breakage. Bleomycin is hydrolyzed by

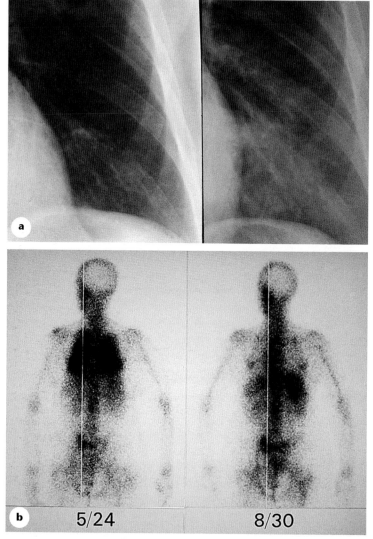

Fig. 5.8 Organ toxicity. Non-mucocutaneous toxicity of chemotherapeutic agents is covered in the text. The lung may be affected by several agents including bleomycin. (a) The earliest radiographic changes are linear infiltrates in the lower lung fields. (b) Gallium-67 uptake is quite striking but is reversible, as this serial study demonstrates.

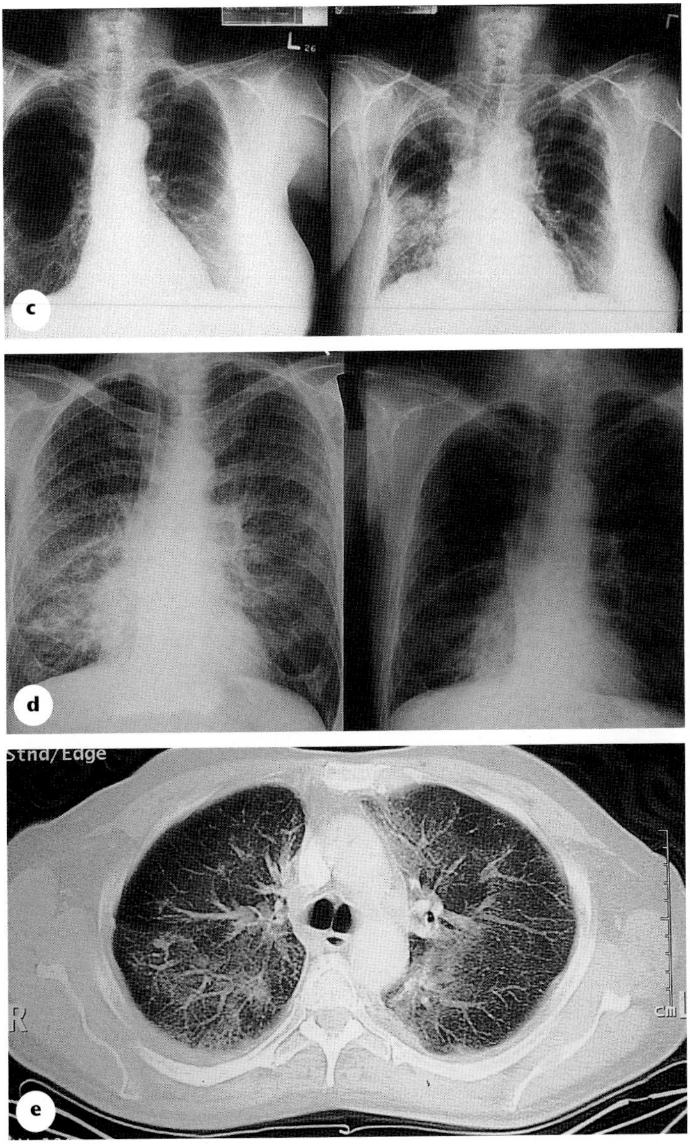

Fig. 5.8 *Continued* (**c**) While usually dose related, progressive changes may occur resulting in fibrosis and pulmonary insufficiency. Other drugs such as alkylating agents and high-dose methotrexate may result in diffuse infiltrates (**d**), which were reversible 4 months later. (**e**) In this patient several courses of gemcitabine resulted in acute dyspnoea and decreased oxygen saturation. Evaluation with lung biopsy and other studies showed no evidence of infection, pulmonary emboli or other diagnosable disease. Use of prednisone led to rapid improvement and regression of the interstitial infiltrates.

bleomycin hydrolase, a cysteine present in normal and malignant cells but decreased in lung and skin.

Busulfan, mitomycin C and carmustine are direct-acting alkylating agents that can cause chronic interstitial pneumonitis and fibrosing alveolitis. This chronic fibrosis produces the clinical picture of progressive, often fatal, restrictive lung disease. The symptoms occur insidiously, often after prolonged therapy. The chronic use of busulfan for the treatment of chronic myelogenous leukaemia is now a historical footnote but carmustine remains the mainstay of treatment for glioblastoma and anaplastic astrocytomas. Cyclophosphamide has been implicated in chronic pulmonary toxicity but rarely as a single agent, more often after radiation.

The antimetabolite methotrexate may produce an acute eosinophilic pneumonitis, which represents an allergic reaction. Cytosine arabinoside and gemcitabine (2',2'-difluoro-2'-deoxycytidine) may also cause an acute pneumonitis, which may be fatal if unrecognized. In these circumstances, withdrawal of the offending agent, supportive care and corticosteroids may prevent a fatal outcome.[12] Some of the reported pulmonary syndromes associated with chemotherapy drugs are noted in Table 5.1.

Table 5.1 Pulmonary syndromes associated with specific cancer chemotherapy drugs

Syndrome	Associated cancer chemotherapy drugs
Pulmonary capillary leak	Interleukin-2, recombinant tumour necrosis factor alpha, cytarabine, mitomycin
Asthma	Interleukin-2, vinca alkaloids plus mitomycin
Bronchiolitis obliterans organizing pneumonia	Bleomycin, cyclophosphamide, methotrexate, mitomycin
Hypersensitivity pneumonitis	Busulfan, bleomycin, etoposide, methotrexate, mitomycin, procarbazine
Interstitial pneumonia/fibrosis	Bleomycin, busulfan, chlorambucil, cyclophosphamide, melphalan, methotrexate, nitrosureas, procarbazine, vinca alkaloids (with mitomycin), gefitinib, erlotinib
Pleural effusion	Bleomycin, busulfan, interleukin-2, methotrexate, mitomycin, procarbazine
Pulmonary vascular injury	Busulfan, nitrosureas

Adapted with permission from Belknap SM, Kuzel TM, Yarnold PR, et al: Clinical features and correlates of gemcitabine-associated lung injury. Cancer 2006; 106: 2051–2057

Both erlotinib and gefitinib, new oral agents targeted at the epidermal growth factor receptor 1, both have a low (<1%) but real incidence of interstitial pneumonitis that resolves if the agent is stopped. The highest incidence is in Asian patients, where 3.5% of patients may develop interstitial disease also referred to as ground glass opacities, which carries a mortalilty of 1.6%.[13]

HEPATOTOXICITY

The liver is a frequent organ for toxicity with cancer chemotherapeutic agents. Centrilobular hepatocyte injury is the frequent histological finding, elevated transaminases the biochemical manifestation. Antimetabolite drugs such as cytosine arabinoside, methotrexate, hydroxycarbamide and 6-Mercaptopurine are all associated with hepatic injury. 6-Mercaptopurine produces a cholestatic picture, with an elevated alkaline phosphatase and bilirubin. L-Asparaginase and carmustine cause hepatotoxicity as well. The injury reverses with discontinuation of the drug. Chronic methotrexate administration, such as in the treatment of autoimmune diseases, is associated with irreversible fibrosis and cirrhosis.

Hepatic vascular injury is another type of injury to the liver associated with cancer chemotherapeutic agents. Hepatic veno-occlusive disease may occur in up to 20% of patients receiving high-dose chemotherapy in conjunction with bone marrow transplantation, with a mortality up to 50%. Jaundice, ascites and hepatomegaly are the full manifestations of veno-occlusive disease but right upper quadrant pain and weight gain occur more frequently. Obliteration of the central hepatic venules and resulting pressure necrosis of the hepatocytes is seen at autopsy. Many regimens and many individual drugs have been implicated. With busulfan, adjustment of the plasma concentration–time profile may reduce the risk. Dacarbazine, a monofunctional alkylating agent, may produce an eosinophilic centrilobular injury with hepatic vein thromboses.

GASTROINTESTINAL TOXICITY

Chemotherapy-induced diarrhoea has been described with several drugs including the fluoropyrimidines (particularly 5-FU), irinotecan, methotrexate and cisplatin. However, it is the major toxicity of regimens containing a fluoropyrimidine and/or irinotecan that can be dose limiting. Both 5-FU and irinotecan cause acute damage to the intestinal mucosa, leading to loss of epithelium. 5-FU causes a mitotic arrest of crypt cells, leading to an increase in the ratio of immature secretory crypt cells to mature villous enterocytes. The increased volume of fluid that leaves the small bowel exceeds the absorptive capacity of the colon, leading to clinically significant diarrhoea.

In patients treated with irinotecan, early-onset diarrhoea, which occurs during or within several hours of drug infusion in 45–50% of patients, is cholinergically mediated. This effect is thought to be due to structural similarity with acetylcholine. In contrast, late irinotecan-associated diarrhoea is not cholinergically mediated. The pathophysiology of late diarrhoea appears to be multifactorial with contributions from dysmotility and secretory factors as well as a direct toxic effect of the drug on the intestinal mucosa.

Irinotecan produces mucosal changes associated with apoptosis, such as epithelial vacuolization, and goblet cell hyperplasia, suggestive of mucin hypersecretion. These changes appear to be related to the accumulation of the active metabolite of irinotecan, SN-38, in the intestinal mucosa. SN-38 is glucuronidated in the liver and is then excreted in the bile. The conjugated metabolite SN-38G does not appear to cause diarrhoea. However, SN-38G can be deconjugated in the intestines by β-glucuronidase present in intestinal bacteria. A direct correlation has been noted between mucosal damage and either low glucuronidation rates or increased intestinal β-glucuronidase activity. Severe toxicity has been described following irinotecan therapy in patients with Gilbert's syndrome, who have defective hepatic glucuronidation. Experimental studies have shown that inhibition of intestinal β-glucuronidase activity with antibiotics protects against mucosal injury and ameliorates the diarrhoea.

Several recently approved receptor tyrosine kinase inhibitors have diarrhoea associated with use, including sorafenib, sunitinib, erlotinib and gefitinib. The frequency varies from 30–40% with less than 5% grade 3 (severe).[14] Also, rare cases of gastrointestinal perforation have been reported using new agents with several mechanisms of action, including inhibitors of tumour vasculature.[15] Hypertension and rare strokes are also side effects that have been reported.

NEUROTOXICITY

Neurotoxicity from cancer chemotherapeutic agents is an increasingly recognized consequence of cancer treatment. The toxicities observed may affect the brain and spinal cord (CNS), peripheral nerves or the supporting neurological tissues such as the meninges. Neurotoxicity from cancer therapeutic drugs must be distinguished from the effects of space-occupying metastatic lesions, toxic metabolic effects from disorders of blood chemistry, adjunctive drugs (such as opiate narcotics) and paraneoplastic syndromes. Toxicity may be acute, subacute or chronic, reversible or irreversible.

The direct-acting alkylating agents ifosfamide and carmustine cause somnolence, confusion and coma at high doses. The toxicity of ifosfamide is secondary to accumulation of a metabolite, chlorethyl aldehyde, in cerebrospinal fluid. Renal dysfunction may cause CNS toxicity at low doses when acidosis results in increased chlorethyl aldehyde levels.

Damage from the antimetabolite methotrexate occurs in three forms and is worse when given intrathecally with radiation. Chemical arachnoiditis, characterized by headache, fever and nuchal rigidity, is the most common and most acute toxicity. This may be due to additives in the diluent (benzoic acid in sterile water). Subacute toxicity is delayed for 2–3 weeks after administration and is characterized by extremity motor paralysis, cranial nerve palsy seizures and coma. This is due to prolonged exposure to high doses of methotrexate. Chronic demyelinating encephalitis produces dementia and spasticity. There is cortical thinning with enlarged ventricles and cerebral calcifications. Types 2 and 3 may be increased after irradiation especially if concomitant systemic therapy with high (or intermediate) doses is used.

Cytosine arabinoside, when given at high doses, produces cerebral and cerebellar dysfunction due to Purkinje cell necrosis and damage. At standard doses, leukoencephalopathy occurs rarely. When given intrathecally, cytosine arabinoside can produce transverse myelitis with resulting paralysis. 5-FU may produce acute cerebellar toxicity due to inhibition of acontinase, an enzyme in the cerebellar Krebs cycle. The purine adenine deaminase inhibitors pentostatin and fludarabine may produce several types of neurotoxicity. Pentostatin produces somnolence and coma at high doses. Fludarabine may cause delayed-onset coma or cortical blindness at high doses, peripheral neuropathy at low doses. Peripheral neuropathy is a frequent toxicity encountered with many cancer chemotherapeutic agents of many classes. Cisplatin and oxaliplatin, the vinca alkaloids and the taxanes all produce peripheral neuropathy in a cumulative dose-dependent manner (see p.73-76 for more on oxaliplatin-related neurotoxicity).

NEPHROTOXICITY

One of the most serious side-effects of chemotherapeutic agents is nephrotoxicity. Any part of the kidney structure (e.g. the glomerulus, the tubules, the interstitium or the renal microvasculature) could be vulnerable to damage. The clinical manifestations of nephrotoxicity can range from an asymptomatic elevation of serum creatinine to acute renal failure requiring dialysis. Intravascular volume depletion secondary to ascites, oedema or external losses, concomitant use of nephrotoxic drugs, urinary tract obstruction secondary to the underlying malignancy, tumour infiltration of the kidney and intrinsic renal disease can potentiate renal dysfunction in the cancer patient.

Platinum compounds are the agents most associated with renal toxicity. Cisplatin is one of the most commonly used and effective chemotherapeutic agents available and also the best studied antineoplastic nephrotoxic drug. It is a potent tubular toxin, particularly in a low chloride environment, such as the interior of cells. Cell death results via apoptosis or necrosis as DNA-damaged cells enter the cell cycle. Approximately 25–35% of patients will develop a mild and partially reversible decline in renal function after the first course of therapy. The incidence and severity of renal failure increase with subsequent courses, eventually becoming in part irreversible. As a result, discontinuing therapy is generally indicated in those patients who develop a progressive rise in plasma creatinine concentration. In addition to this rise, potentially irreversible hypomagnesaemia due to urinary magnesium wasting may occur in over one-half of cases.

There is suggestive evidence that the nephrotoxicity of cisplatin can be diminished by vigorous hydration and perhaps by giving the drug in a hypertonic solution. A high chloride concentration may minimize both the formation of the highly reactive platinum compounds described above and the uptake of cisplatin by the renal tubular cells. Amifostine, an organic thiophosphate, appears to diminish cisplatin-induced toxicity by donating a protective thiol group, an effect that is highly selective for normal, but not malignant, tissue. Discontinuation of platinum therapy once the plasma creatinine concentration begins to rise should prevent progressive renal failure.

Carboplatin has been synthesized as a non-nephrotoxic platinum analogue, but even though it is less nephrotoxic, it is not free of potential for renal injury. Hypomagnesaemia appears to be the most common manifestation of nephrotoxicity. Other, less common renal side-effects include recurrent salt wasting. No significant clinical nephrotoxicity due to oxaliplatin has yet been reported. Limited data have shown no exacerbation of pre-existing mild renal impairment. Studies of oxaliplatin in patients with progressive degrees of renal failure are in progress.

Cyclophosphamide may produce significant side-effects involving the urinary bladder (haemorrhagic cystitis). The primary renal effect of this agent is hyponatraemia, which is due to impairment of the ability of the kidney to excrete water. The mechanism appears to be due to a direct effect of cyclophosphamide on the distal tubule and not to increased levels of antidiuretic hormone. Hyponatraemia usually occurs acutely and resolves upon discontinuation of the drug (approximately 24 hours). It is recommended that isotonic saline be infused prior to cyclophosphamide administration in order to ameliorate this effect.

Ifosfamide nephrotoxicity has a primary renal effect to produce tubular renal toxicity. The damage produced by ifosfamide is concentrated in the proximal renal tubule and a Fanconi syndrome has been observed after therapy. Other clinical syndromes that have been associated with ifosfamide include nephrogenic diabetes insipidus, renal tubular acidosis and rickets. Pre-existing renal disease is an important risk factor for ifosfamide nephrotoxicity.

Carmustine, lomustine and semustine are lipid-soluble nitrosureas, which have been used against brain tumours. The exact mechanism of nephrotoxicity, however, is incompletely understood. High doses of semustine in children and adults have been associated with progressive renal dysfunction to marked renal insufficiency 3–5 years after therapy. The characteristic histological changes include glomerular sclerosis without immune deposits and interstitial fibrosis. The incidence of nephrotoxicity was reported at 26% in patients with malignant melanoma treated with methyl CCNU in the adjuvant setting. Nephrotoxicity has been reported in 65–75% of patients treated with streptozotocin for prolonged periods of time. Proteinuria is often the first sign of renal damage. This is followed by signs of proximal tubular damage, such as phosphaturia, glycosuria, aminoaciduria, uricosuria and bicarbonaturia. Renal toxicity lasts approximately 2–3 weeks after discontinuing the drug.

The most common form of nephrotoxicity associated with mitomycin C is haemolytic uraemic syndrome. It has been reported in patients who were treated with total doses of mitomycin C in excess of 60 mg/m^2. The renal damage caused by this antineoplastic agent appears to be direct endothelial damage. The incidence of this syndrome ranges from 4% to 6% of patients who receive this drug alone or in combination.

Low or standard doses of methotrexate are usually not associated with renal toxicity, unless patients have underlying renal dysfunction. High doses (1–15 g/m^2) are associated with a 47% incidence of renal toxicity, accompanied by methotrexate crystals in the urine. The mechanism for methotrexate-induced nephrotoxicity is explained in part by its limited solubility at an acid pH, which leads to intratubular precipitation. Patients who are volume depleted and excrete an acidic urine are at higher risk for nephrotoxicity. With aggressive hydration and urine alkalinization, the incidence of renal failure with high doses of methotrexate can be decreased. The clinical picture of methotrexate-induced renal failure is that of a non-oliguric renal failure. Preventive measures when using high doses of methotrexate include aggressive intravenous hydration with saline and urine alkalinization with sodium bicarbonate to maintain a urine pH around 7.0. If renal failure develops, methotrexate levels will increase and the risk of systemic toxicity will also be enhanced. In addition to supportive measures, patients should be started on folinic acid rescue, until levels of methotrexate fall below 0.5 uM.

VEGF or VEGFR2-targeted agents produce albuminuria in 10–25% of patients, sometimes to nephrotic range. The exact mechanism has not been elucidated but studies in mice with conditional expression of VEGF in the podocytes confirms a major role for VEGF in endothelial development and maintainence of a fenestrated endothelium.[16] Like hypertension, this appears to be a class effect but the factors associated with occurrence and severity are unknown. If clinically significant, decreasing the dose or discontinuation of drug are the only current approaches.

LATE COMPLICATIONS OF CANCER CHEMOTHERAPY

As cancer therapy has become increasingly effective and more patients live longer, late complications have become apparent separate from the direct toxic effects on organ system function described above. Gonadal dysfunction is one. In males, the primary lesion is depletion of germinal epithelium of seminiferous tubules with marked decrease in testicular volume, oligo- or azoospermia and infertility. There is an increase in follicle-stimulating hormone (FSH) and occasionally in luteinizing hormone (LH). No change is seen in serum testosterone. Alkylating agents (and irradiation) are the most damaging and toxicity is dose related. About 80% of males with Hodgkin's disease treated with MOPP are oligo-azoospermic. About half recover in up to 4 years. Procarbazine is a major offender. Anthracyclines also cause azoospermia in a dose-related fashion. In females, the primary lesion is ovarian fibrosis and follicle destruction. Amenorrhoea ensues, with increase in FSH and LH and a decrease in oestradiol leading to vaginal atrophy and endometrial hypoplasia. Onset and duration are dose and age related. Alkylating agents (and irradiation) again are the worst offenders.

In children, the prepubertal effects may be less profound and reversible in males, though the pubertal effects may be more severe with often irreversible azoospermia, decreased testosterone and increased FSH and LH. Less is known about females, but young girls appear quite resistant to alkylating agents.

No more tragic toxicity is seen with cancer chemotherapeutic agents than the induction of a second, treatment-related cancer in a patient cured of one cancer.[17,18] Of the wide variety of environmental and chemical agents causing cancer, there is one common thread in their mode of action – interaction with DNA. Clinical studies detailing this consequence of therapy have many problems, including the inherent bias of reporting index cases, the retrospective nature of many reports, the lack of reliable information on drug dosage, total amount of drug given and duration of therapy and the underlying incidence of second malignancy. The direct-acting alkylating agents are most often implicated and chronic, low-dose administration is a greater risk factor. Acute non-lymphocytic leukaemia or myelodysplasia is the best described. The indirect-acting topoisomerase II agents produce a specific 11q23 translocation.

Osteonecrosis of the jaw has been seen with increasing frequency during the past few years, related in part to chronic use of intravenous bisphophonates for advanced cancer. The incidence has been estimated at 1–10% of patients receiving these medications.[19] The pathogenesis and optimal management for osteonecrosis of the jaw are poorly understood, with multiple risk factors and various treatments involved.[20]

REFERENCES

1. Weiss RB: Toxicity of chemotherapy – the last decade. Semin Oncol 2006; 33: 1.
2. Crawford J, Cella D, Sonis ST: Managing chemotherapy-related side effects: trends in the use of cytokines and other growth factors. Oncology 2006; 20: Suppl.
3. Zorzou MP, Efstathiou E, Galani E, et al: Carboplatin hypersensitivity reactions. J Chemother 2005; 17(1): 104–110.
4. Cristaaudo A, Sera F, Severino V, et al: Occupational hypersensitivity to metal salts, including platinum, in the secondary industry. Allergy 2005; 60(2): 138–139.
5. Szebeni J: Complement activation-related pseudoallergy: a new class of drug induced acute immune toxicity. Toxicology 2005; 216: 106–121.
6. Escudier B, Szczylik C, Eisen T, et al: Randomized phase III trial of the Raf kinase and VEGFR inhibitor sorafenib (BAY 43-9006) in patients with advanced renal cell carcinoma (RCC). J Clin Oncol 2005; 23(18 Suppl): abstract 4510.
7. Perez-Solar R, Saltz L. Cutaneous adverse effects with HER1/EGFR-targeted agents: is there a silver lining? J Clin Oncol 2005; 23(24): 5235–5246.
8. Floyd JD, Nguyen DT, Lobins RL, et al: Cardiotoxicity of cancer therapy. J Clin Oncol 2005; 23: 7685–7696.

9. Kerkela R, Grazette L, Yacobi R, et al: Cardiotoxicity of the cancer therapeutic agent imatinib mesylate. Nat Med 2006; 12(8): 908–916.

10. Hurwitz H: Integrating the anti-VEGF – A humanized monoclonal antibody bevacizumab with chemotherapy in advanced colorectal cancer. Clin Colorectal Cancer 2004; 4 Suppl 2: S62–S68.

11. Motzer RJ, Hutson TE, Tomczak P, et al: Phase III randomized trial of sunitinib malate (SU11248) versus interferon alfa as first line systemic therapy for patients with metastatic renal cell carcinoma. J Clin Oncol 2006; 24 (18 Suppl): 930s abstract LBA3.

12. Belknap SM, Kuzel TM, Yarnold PR, et al: Clinical features and correlates of gemcitabine-associated lung injury. Cancer 2006; 106: 2051–2057.

13. Ando M, Okamoto I, Yamamoto N, et al: Predictive factors for interstitial lung disease, antitumor response, and survival in non-small-cell lung cancer patients treated with gefitinib. J Clin Oncol 2006; 24: 2549–2556.

14. Niho S, Kubota K, Goto K, et al: First-line single agent treatment with gefitinib in patients with advanced non-small cell lung cancer: a phase II study. J Clin Oncol 2006; 24(1): 64–69.

15. Ratain MJ, Eisen T, Stadler WM, et al: Phase II placebo-controlled randomized discontinuation trial of sorafenib in patients with metastatic renal cell carcinoma. J Clin Oncol 2006; 24: 2505–2512.

16. Erimina V, Quaggin SE: The role of VEGF-A in glomerular development and function. Curr Opin Nephrol Hypertens 2004; 13: 9–15.

17. Bhatia S, Landier W: Evaluating survivors of pediatric cancer. Cancer J 2005; 11: 340–354.

18. Hudson MM, Mertens AC, Yasui Y, et al: Health status in adults treated for childhood cancer: a report from the childhood survivor study. Am J Oncol Rev 2004; 3: 165–170.

19. Badros A, Weikel D, Salama A, et al: Osteonecrosis of the jaw in multiple myeloma patients: clinical features and risk factors. J Clin Oncol 2006; 24: 945–952.

20. Ruggiero S, Gralow J, Marx RE, et al. Practical guidelines for the prevention, diagnosis and treatment of osteonecrosis of the jaw in patients with cancer. J Oncol Pract 2006; 2: 7–14.

FURTHER READING

Adrian RM, Hood, AF, Skarin AT. Mucocutaneous reactions to antineoplastic agents. CA Cancer J Clin 1980; 30: 143–157.

Attar EC, Ervin T, Janicek M, Deykin A, Godleski J: Acute interstitial pneumonitis related to gemcitabine. J Clin Oncol 2000; 18: 697–698.

Burstein H: Radiation recall dermatitis from gemcitabine. J Clin Oncol 2000; 18: 693–694.

Chabner BA, Longo DL: Cancer Chemotherapy and Biotherapy, 2nd edn. Lippincott–Raven, Philadelphia, 1996.

Darnell J, Lodish H, Baltimore D: Molecular Cell Biology, 3rd edn. W.H. Freeman, New York, 1995.

DeVita VT, Jr, Hellman S, Rosenberg SA: Cancer: Principles and Practice of Oncology, 4th edn. Lippincott, Philadelphia, 1993.

Eder JP: Neoplasms. In: Page CP, Curtis MJ, Sutter MC, Walker MJA, Hoffman BB, eds: Integrated Pharmacology. Mosby–Times Mirror International, London, 1997: 501–522.

Hussain S, Anderson DN, Salvatti ME, et al: Onycholysis as a complication of systemic chemotherapy. Cancer 2000; 88: 2367–2371.

Perry MD: The Chemotherapy Source Book. Williams and Wilkins, Baltimore, 1992.

Skeel RT: Handbook of Cancer Chemotherapy. Little, Brown, Boston, 1991.

Sonis ST, Fey EG: Oral complications of cancer therapy. Oncology 2002; 16: 680–691.

Index